GOVERNORS STATE UNIVERSITY LIBRARY

3 1611 00237 5852

GOVERNORS STATE UNIVERSITY
LIBRA

D1517498

DEMCO

MEDICINE IN THE DAYS OF THE PHARAOHS

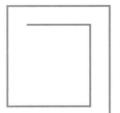

MEDICINE
IN THE DAYS OF THE PHARAOHS

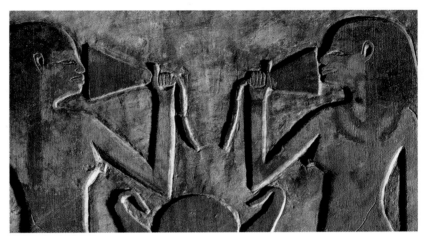

Bruno Halioua

Translated by M. B. DeBevoise

Bernard Ziskind

GOVERNORS STATE UNIVERSITY
UNIVERSITY PARK
IL 60466

THE BELKNAP PRESS OF HARVARD UNIVERSITY PRESS

Cambridge, Massachusetts, and London, England   2005

R
137
.H3413
2005

Copyright © 2005 by the President and Fellows of Harvard College
All rights reserved
Printed in the United States of America
Originally published as *La médecine au temps des pharaons;*
  © Éditions Liana Levi, 2002

Library of Congress Cataloging-in-Publication Data

Halioua, Bruno, 1959–
    [Médecine au temps des pharaons. English]
    Medicine in the days of the pharaohs / Bruno Halioua and Bernard Ziskind ;
translated by M. B. DeBevoise.
        p. cm.
    Includes bibliographical references and index.
    ISBN 0-674-01702-1
    1. Medicine, Egyptian.   I. Title.

R137.H3413 2005   2004057367
610'.932—dc22

Contents

Endmatter

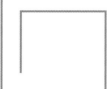

Donald B. Redford

Foreword

The last half century has witnessed an astonishing increase in our knowledge of ancient Egypt, thanks not only to an increased number of research expeditions but also to improvement in archaeological method and theory and the application of new models and techniques drawn from anthropology and the hard sciences. In no field has that advance in knowledge been greater than in medicine and pathology. In fact it has become almost de rigueur to number a physician or pathologist among the field staff of any archaeological expedition, and not only those excavating ancient burial grounds. The intensity of this research interest has given rise over the past four decades to a series of autopsies on mummies and other human remains, both those long resident in museums and those newly excavated in the field, using the most up-to-date techniques, both intrusive and non-intrusive.

A like interest has long been directed toward what the ancient Egyptians themselves had to say about the medicine they practiced. About ten medical compendia in papyrus form are extant, spanning nearly three millennia in time. In fact, as is the case in the history of many communities newly arrived from a prehistoric stage of sociopolitical evolution, it was the medical lore and the pharmacopoeia that were among the first words to be committed to visible speech in that newfangled invention, writing. Later tradition is insistent upon crediting the earliest kings of Egypt with being the authors of medical treatises.

The present book is the latest in a time-honored sequence of modern works on the theory and practice of Egyptian medicine, and it takes its place as one of the most authoritative and clearly written. When in a discipline the primary, scientific reports of research begin to proliferate rapidly, an overarching synthesis is desperately required by both student and scholar, and that is just what Messrs. Halioua and Ziskind have provided. The authors pay attention, not only to the results of archaeology and forensic investigation, but also to the ancient texts, which they quote extensively, and the constant reference to these original sources makes the reader acutely aware of the limitations of our primary evidence. In particular we sometimes forget, if we are not familiar with the ancient language, how little known are the terms used by ancient Egyptian doctors for the diseases they had to cure, the medical implements they used, and the drugs they prescribed. The authors do not dwell narrowly on medical practice as such, but broaden their account to include practitioners and patients within a socioeconomic context. Bewildering, perhaps, for us moderns is the fact that in many passages of the ancient books of medicine sober and informed observation and diagnosis are found side by side with what many of us would pass off as "magical nonsense." It is to the authors' credit that they adopt an unprejudiced scholarly approach to this implicit belief in the power of magic, which characterizes ancient Egypt to a greater extent than most other Old World cultures. Readers will also be grateful for the inclusion of evidence derived from the very latest research being undertaken in the field of the paleopathology of mummies. For those whose only brush with the ancient land of the Nile has been by way of Bible stories about Joseph and Moses and Israel in Egypt, there is an extended disquisition on the Ten Plagues recounted in the Book of Exodus. Finally, the addition of an extensive bibliography will be a boon for both lay reader and scholar alike, and will win the heartfelt thanks of those wishing to advance further in the study of ancient Egyptian medicine.

To the translator we owe a deep debt of gratitude for a highly successful rendering in English which does not slavishly parrot the original, but by careful and judicious redaction on a minor scale serves the reader of English well. Translations often lose a certain element of power and immediacy because of the necessary adaptation to a new lexical range. But this work is one of the exceptions, for the product flows easily with novel turns of phrase, yet maintains precision and accuracy.

Alike for those mesmerized by the mysterious world of Egyptian medicine and those who enter into it with scholarly intent, this book encompasses it all in a well-ordered and accurate manner. Reader, enjoy! You are in for a rewarding experience.

—Donald B. Redford
Pennsylvania State University

Translator's Note

Complete consistency is not in the nature of things Egyptological, as John Ray has observed, and so with regard to the spelling of personal and place names some arbitrariness is unavoidable. I have tried to follow the example of the *Oxford History of Ancient Egypt* in this connection and also, more generally, the modern tendency to run syllables together rather than separating them (thus, for example, Ankhmahor rather than Ankh-ma-hor). In compensation for the loss of so many familiar hyphens I have taken the liberty of dispensing with the various diacritical marks customarily employed by Egyptologists, which they will not miss and other readers do not need to see.

In textual matters I have on the whole respected Bardinet's landmark translation of the medical corpus, which builds upon—and in places supersedes—the monumental nine-volume *Grundriss der Medizin der alten Ägypter* by Grapow, von Deines, and Westendorf. In the case of the Ebers and Edwin Smith papyri I have compared Bardinet's renderings with those of Ebbell and Breasted, as well as the ones given by Nunn in his recent work on ancient Egyptian medicine, and have occasionally made small modifications to the French text. Where a substantive point is at issue I have described it in a note.

For the sake of readability I have eliminated some of Bardinet's embedded glosses and simplified his elaborate system of bracketed interpolations. With regard to the transliteration of medical terms and names of ancient Egyptian practitioners I have frequently, though not always, preferred Nunn's readings. Since there is no generally accepted convention for the translation of physicians' titles I have also, where possible, included the Egyptian terms in the text and marked variant readings in the notes.

Finally, I have compiled a bibliography from the notes to the French edition, adding to it a number of works that proved to be useful in preparing the English translation. I am grateful to Ian Shaw for his comments on a draft of the translation, and to the staff of several libraries at Tulane University for research assistance.

—M. B. DeBevoise

MEDICINE IN THE DAYS OF THE PHARAOHS

Introduction

The renewed interest in history that has come with the ending of one century and the beginning of another is a sign that societies need time to reflect about the past. It is particularly pronounced in a field such as medicine, where major changes have taken place. Many people, practitioners and patients alike, wish to have a basis for comparison and explanation. The history of medicine, long neglected by practitioners themselves, provides an excellent opportunity for understanding the problems that physicians face in their daily practice, as the historian Charles Lichtenthaeler has rightly sought to impress upon students: professional knowledge by itself merely produces technical experts, health functionaries; real stature in the practice of medicine requires historical awareness.[1]

But why take a special interest in Egyptian medicine? There is, first of all, the fascination exerted by ancient Egypt as the source of the Western spiritual tradition. Albert Champdor well described this attraction in his introduction to *The Book of the Dead:* "One has only to set foot in Egypt to recognize at once the presence of a marvelous civilization, to accept it as the gift of vanished generations. Egypt, six thousand years old, immediately welcomes you and enchants you." This fascination is hardly new: in antiquity a great many philosophers were strongly influenced by their travels in the land of the eternal river. The thought of Homer, Plato, Pythagoras, Plutarch, Thales, Herodotus, and Solon was shaped to a considerable degree by Egyptian culture. Their writings established a continuity between Egyptian and Western civilization—interrupted by the burning of the library at Alexandria and the closing of the pagan temples of the Roman Empire by Theodosius in A.D. 391. With the demise of these shrines, at a time when hieroglyphic writing had all but disappeared, the last traces of ancient Egypt were lost. During the fourteen centuries that followed, Egyptian civilization fell further into oblivion, as its architectural treasures endured the throes of successive occupations and its literary, artistic, and scientific achievements were forgotten.[2]

It was not until Egyptian writing yielded up its secrets to Jean-François Champollion in 1822 that this marvelous culture was rediscovered and the discipline of Egyptology was born, along with a mania for all things Egyptian. Subsequent research has revealed the avant-garde character of Egyptian civilization, which made original contributions in the domains of astrology, architecture, geometry, and medicine. Yet even after Champollion's breakthrough Egyptian medical thought remained almost completely unknown. So great was the absence of documentary evidence, and so faint the memory of more ancient accomplishments, that the origin of Western medicine was unanimously attributed to the legendary figure of Hippocrates.

Some twenty-five centuries before the Greek "father of medicine" laid the foundations of modern medicine, there already existed a coherent and largely codified body of practice that indisputably influenced the medical thought of the Hebrews, the Greeks, and the Romans. Yet it was only toward the end of the nineteenth century of our era, with the discovery and translation of papyri that incorporated a mixture of medical and magical elements, that scholarly interest in Egyptian medicine really began to develop. The first transcriptions had the disadvantage, however, of being only approximate, both lessening and distorting the appreciation these treatises deserved. Indeed, they gave rise to a lasting misconception, namely that Egyptian medicine amounted to nothing more than a medico-magical compendium devoid of objective scientific value.

This misconception gave rise in turn to lively debate among scholars of Egyptian medicine. On one side were enthusiasts, such as Naguib Riad, who saw it as a genuine science unrivaled by any contemporary tradition. On the other were more moderate proponents, such as Henry E. Sigerist, Frans Jonckheere, and Ange Pierre Leca, who sought to bring out the complexity of an art of healing that was variously magical and religious, empirical and rational, depending on the case. The metic-

A statue of Imhotep, who during the 3rd Dynasty served as royal chamberlain, high priest of Heliopolis, and architect of the pharaoh Djoser's pyramid at Saqqara. He was later deified and, in his role as patron of scribes and physicians, identified with Asclepius, the Greek god of medicine. Though it is not known whether Imhotep held the title of *swnw*, some authorities regard him as the first physician of the ancient world, anticipating Hippocrates by more than two millennia. He is shown here holding a papyrus roll, symbolic of wisdom. Museum of Fine Arts, Boston.

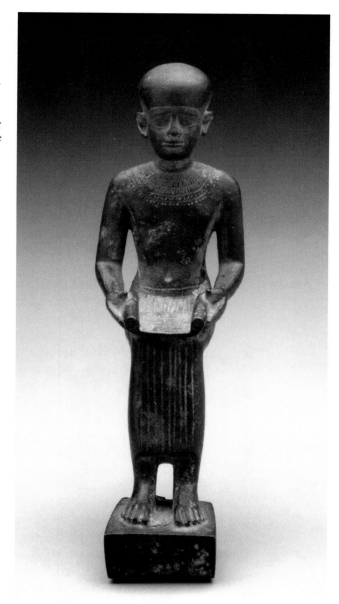

ulous translation of the medical papyri—first by Walter Wreszinski, and then by James Henry Breasted, Bendix Ebbell, Erik Iversen, John W. B. Barns, Hermann Grapow, Hildegard von Deines, and Wolfhart Westendorf, and above all Thierry Bardinet—has permitted greater insight into the nature of illnesses in ancient Egypt and the manner in which they were treated. The past three decades have witnessed extraordinary breakthroughs in paleopathology and remarkable progress in the domain of Egyptology generally, marked by improved understanding of hieroglyphic scripts and the discovery of several texts whose challenge to received wisdom has stimulated research in the fields of epidemiology, pathology, and therapeutics.

Our own interest in the medicine of the days of the pharaohs came about in a wholly fortuitous way. Celebrating the festival of Passover, we were required by tradition to explain to our children the "ten plagues of Egypt." It was our inability to give a definite answer to the question of what caused the death of the Egyptian firstborn children that led us to take a passionate interest in this neglected chapter in the history of medicine. A sizable literature exists on most aspects of Egyptian civilization, but until recently there has been comparatively little on medicine. Our training enabled us to appreciate the skill of pharaonic physicians. They were not mere bonesetters who relied mainly on psychology, as certain authors having no knowledge of medicine wrongly maintain.

The present work therefore aims to help fill a gap. Above all, however, we wish to communicate our admiration for Egyptian medicine, to which today's practitioners are indebted in their daily exercise of the art of Asclepius—or rather, as one should say, of Imhotep. In examining the medical papyri we have tried to survey the full extent of Egyptian knowledge. Remarkably, the medicine practiced in ancient Egypt remained roughly the same throughout the three millennia during which the pharaohs reigned.

Studying illness and disease in the context of daily life makes it possible, we believe, to approach pharaonic civilization from a particularly illuminating perspective—sharing as we do the view of another historian of medicine, Erwin H. Ackerknecht, that "the pathology of a society reflects its general conditions and its development, and thus furnishes information that is useful for understanding the society as a whole."[3]

PART I

THE WORLD OF THE PHYSICIAN

1   The Medical Profession

Medical practice in ancient Egypt may be compared to the kind that existed in France in the nineteenth century, when physicians were distinguished on the one hand from *officiers de santé,* who were authorized to practice without an academic degree, and on the other from bonesetters (sometimes called *guérisseurs,* or healers). These figures find approximate equivalents in the three representatives of the medical profession in pharaonic Egypt mentioned in the Ebers papyrus (854a): "If any doctor *(swnw),* any priest *(wab)* of Sekhmet, or any magician *(sau)* places his two hands or his fingers on the head, on the back of the head, on the hands, on the place of the heart . . ." Some commentators believe that the term *swnw* (plural *swnww*) designated "the secular physician par excellence," by contrast with the *wab*-priest of the warrior goddess Sekhmet, who was considered a healer, and the *kherep*-priest of the scorpion goddess Serqet, a charmer (or conjurer of spells) who was regarded wholly as a magician.[1]

This variety of expertise was a natural consequence of the conception of medicine in ancient Egypt. The Egyptians thought of a person suffering from disease or pain as the victim of a negative force, a hostile divinity, indeed of a demon. The purpose of the physician was therefore to combat the invisible and irrational power that disturbed the sick person by reciting either magical formulas or religious incantations.

It was only gradually, as certain remedies proved their effectiveness, that the scientific and rational aspect of medicine asserted itself. Religion nonetheless was the soil out of which science developed. For almost thirty-five hundred years religion regulated the daily life of society, from the pharaoh down to the poorest of his subjects, providing "support for the world against chaos."[2] It is not hard to understand why, among the Egyptians—"the most religious of men," according to Herodotus (2.37), and "the first men of the Earth who knew the gods, constructed temples, built altars, and gathered crowds for religious ceremonies," in the opinion of Lucian of Samosata—the gods played very specific roles in the realm of medicine.[3]

Magic, or *heka,* a collection of rites closely linked to a religious dogma whose myths and beliefs it conveyed, was considered to be a genuine science, at once theoretical and experimental. In Egypt, which Erik Hornung has called the "chosen land of magic," *heka* was seen as an indispensable part of the proper functioning of the world, and, like religion, it frequently affected the events of daily life. The pharaoh, it will be recalled, agreed to allow the Jewish people to leave Egypt only after Moses managed to outdo the feats of Egyptian magicians. Far from being an occult practice, as François Daumas pointed out, this science united "the whole set of forces necessary to the protection of life and to its increase," and thus "included medicine even in its rational approach to healing."[4]

Magic was supposed to keep the human body in harmony with the cosmos, so that it could serve as a receptacle for the vital forces that created the universe. More particularly, it was thought to be capable of treating "internal" illnesses such as fractures, wounds, and injuries, themselves regarded as consequences of "immaterial forces, harmful spirits, or divinities associated with evil." The magician-physician, it was believed, possessed a special power. Charged with the care of the "possessed," he had the ability to act on supernatural forces, spirits, and malevolent demons, and treated not so much the consequences as the cause, not so much disease as evil.[5]

But is it therefore necessary, as certain authors believe, to consider religion and magic a constraint on medical development, "a metaphysical obstacle and substitute order"? Is it actually the case that "in a state of social coexistence where the magical conception of an irrational, supernatural, and mythical world reigns, the notion of natural disease disappears or cannot appear"? Egyptian medicine belonged to a phase that Charles Lichtenthaeler calls "archaic" or "oriental." Marked by changes in social organization, the birth of writing (which permitted the

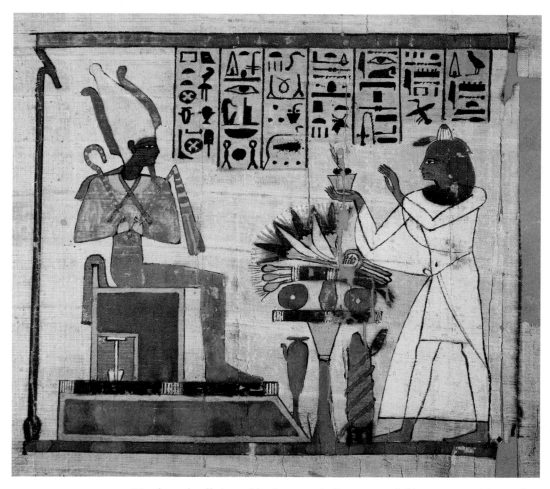

Ritual temple offerings of food were typically accompanied by prayers petitioning the gods of the underworld to grant a long and healthy life (traditionally 110 years) and a prosperous afterlife, and by the burning of incense to purify the burial chamber. Such prayers were first carved on a false door inside tomb-chapels, and later on the coffins holding the dead. This scene, from a papyrus illustrating a coffin text of the 22nd Dynasty, shows Padiamenet, chief baker of the domain of Amun, burning incense for Osiris. British Museum.

recording of advances in theory and clinical practice), and the emergence of the profession of medicine, this phase coincided with the rise of the great empires of antiquity.[6] Medicine in ancient Egypt was from the beginning characterized by two elements, as Dominique Spaeth has argued, "magic being the residue of primitive and tribal thought, rational empiricism the fruit and the contribution of social and cultural development." In the words of Gustave Lefebvre: "Medicine is issued from magic, which is itself only an aspect of religion, and all three, among the Egyptians, remained intimately intermingled with one another."[7]

Physicians and Priests

It was the *swnw* who acted as a physician in our sense of the term. The hieroglyph that designates these practitioners combines three signs: two phonetic elements, an arrow *(swn)* and a vase *(nw),* and the symbol of a seated man, which functions as a determinative.[8] In addition to paintings on the walls of the hypogea, or burial chambers, cut into desert cliffs during the Middle and New Kingdoms, inscriptions discovered on the walls of tombs, on the funerary stelae of physicians themselves, and on those of the high officials to whose service the physicians were attached, as well as on the "false doors," sarcophagi, and statues of funerary chapels, have made it possible to identify some of these figures by name and to reconstruct their careers. The oldest mummy of a physician so far discovered was found very recently, in the autumn of 2001, still intact in its coffin chamber at Saqqara, twenty-one meters below ground: Qa'ar, priest and "chief physician of the secret of the palace," who lived during the 5th Dynasty.[9]

Alongside these *swnww* one finds the *wab*-priests of the dreaded warrior goddess Sekhmet and the exorcists who served the scorpion goddess Serqet. The latter magicians were devoted to more specialized tasks than the *wab*-priests, who, in addition to their duties as physicians, from time to time seem to have dispensed veterinary treatment.[10] As an inscription from the Middle Kingdom found in the alabaster quarries of Hatnub testifies: "I am a priest of Sekhmet, expert in my duties, who puts his hand on the [sick] man and who knows [his illness], who is expert [in the art of] diagnosing with the hand: one who knows oxen . . ." Elsewhere in the quarries a priest of Sekhmet figures in a scene depicting the slaughter of oxen.[11]

The activity of the priestly exorcist has often been defined in opposition to that of the *swnw*, the one figure being characterized by his "sacerdotal character," the other regarded as a civil official. Again, this distinction is not altogether dissimilar to one that existed in France at the time of the Renaissance—between lay and clerical physicians. François Rabelais, a physician who in 1551 became curate of Meudon, combined the two roles.[12]

Gaston Maspero distinguished these two types of practitioners according to their working methods: "The *swnw* is a physician working with reference to books, [whereas] the *wab* of Sekhmet is an ordinary priest, an alchemist, who derives inspiration from his divine mistress, from supernatural formulas." This contrast calls to mind a familiar pair of colleagues in Hippocratic Greece, the inspired healer *(ierus)* and the trained practitioner *(iatros)*. To regard the *wab*-priest of Sekhmet as a member of the medical profession one must be prepared to accept Rémi Picard's intriguing interpretation of a puzzling state of affairs: "The priest of Sekhmet spreads disease and cures it. By appeasing and neutralizing his dangerous mistress, he now becomes her master. Disease being considered a manifestation of Sekhmet, the priest's purity enables him to cure the disease. It is the intervention of the priest of Sekhmet in a medical capacity that makes it possible to consider him a physician."[13]

Complicating matters further is the fact that some figures bear both titles, *swnw* (physician) and *wab* (priest). Thus the funerary stele of Nefer, who practiced under Thutmose I, describes him in these terms: "The priest [of Sekhmet] Nefer says: I am a true physician, skilled with his hands [. . .] sounding the diseases of the body." Thus, too, the stele of Amenhotep states that he exercised the functions of "overseer of the priests of Sekhmet," but his title is "chief of physicians" on the statue dedicated by his son Iuny, himself overseer of the priests of Sekhmet. And Ptahhotep, whose late 5th Dynasty tomb was found at Saqqara, is favored with the dual title "overseer of the priests [of Sekhmet] of the palace, physician."[14] In the New Kingdom all "these magicians [charged] with protecting Egypt and its people against demons and spirits" seem to have been made royal councilors by Rameses II, who awarded them the title of *hery-tep*.[15]

The priests of Serqet constitute a final category. They fall into two classes: *kherep Serqet* ("superiors" or "administrators" of the goddess), of whom some forty are known to us, and *sa Serqet,* who remain in large measure mysterious, the names of scarcely a dozen having been preserved. The scorpion goddess's full name, Serqet-hatyt ("the one who makes the throat breathe," in Frédérique von Känel's translation) evokes her power to cure respiratory disorders caused by venomous bites and stings.[16] Her servants were supposed to be able to prevent and heal injuries due to poisonous serpents and insects by means of medicines and magical formulas: "The one who prepares the way for reviving the dead, for giving air to the blocked nose, for resuscitating the asphyxiated by the movement of his arms as well as by every technique of the *kherep Serqet* . . . the techniques of the *kherep Serqet* [are] used to resuscitate all people, all animals, and to protect them against the venom of all male and female snakes, of all reptiles."[17]

Here again neat categorization is blurred by several figures who bear two or more medical titles: two figures of the 6th Dynasty, Khuy and Irenakhty, are identified as both *swnw* and *kherep Serqet* of the palace.[18] And much later, during the 26th Dynasty, we encounter a man named Psamtek-soneb who was at once chief physician, *kherep Serqet,* and *sa Serqet.*

Medical Specialties

It is natural to look for equivalents of the medical specialties of our own time in the practice of Egyptian physicians. Frans Jonckheere claimed to recognize our surgeon in the *sa hemem* ("man of the cautery"), repeatedly cited in a section of the Ebers papyrus (857–877) dealing with tumors: "Treat it in the same way as a patient of the man of the cautery."[19] But establishing correspondences is not always so simple.

The testimony of Herodotus, a famous visitor to Egypt in about 450 B.C., suggests another way of conceiving the medical profession, namely as one composed almost exclusively of specialists: "The practice of medicine they split up into separate parts, each doctor being responsible for the treatment of only one disease. There are, in consequence, innumerable doctors, some specializing in diseases of the eyes, others of the head, others of the teeth, others of the stomach, and so on; while others, again, deal with the sort of troubles which cannot be exactly localized."[20]

It is possible that Herodotus went too far in generalizing to the medical profession as a whole a situation that may have existed only within the royal palace. But certainly there is evidence of a tendency toward specialization among ordinary physicians long after the pharaonic era. Pliny the Elder, noting the appearance of a contagious skin disease in Italy, first under Tiberius and later under Nero, goes on to say: "There [then] arrived from Egypt, the parent of such diseases, physicians who devoted all their attention to this complaint only." There were other specialists as well, among them ophthalmologists: *swnw irt* (doctor of the eye), *swnw irty* (doctor of the eyes), more rarely *swnw seneb irty* (doctor who heals the two eyes). So great was the renown of these experts that Cyrus, king of Persia, had summoned one of them to his court to cure him of an ocular complaint.[21]

One also finds the equivalents of our dentist: *ibhy* ("one who takes care of the teeth"—from the word for tooth, *ibh*) and *iry ibh* ("one who deals with the teeth"). The difference between these two practitioners is still not very clear. Two *iry ibh* have been identified: Menkawraankh, who practiced during the 5th Dynasty, and Neferirtes, during the Old Kingdom. Among their hierarchical superiors we find mention of a certain Hesyra, a high official at the court of the pharaoh Djoser during the 3rd Dynasty who was styled not only *wer ibhy* ("chief dentist") but also *wer swnw* ("chief physician"). According to Gilles Boulu, Hesyra was probably the "oldest holder of the title *swnw*" and "the first dentist in history."[22]

Another chief of dentists, Khuy, combined this specialty with proctology. In this capacity he was referred to as "guardian of the anus" *(neru pehut)*, a title borne by physicians qualified to prescribe and administer medicines rectally.[23] Herodotus frequently speaks of the alimentary canal: the Egyptians, he says, "purge themselves, for their health's sake, with emetics and clysters." Diodorus Siculus, writing four hundred years later, echoes this observation, saying that "in order to prevent sicknesses they look after the health of their bodies by means of drenches, fastings, and emetics." Enemas were among the most common modes of treatment, employed several times a month for preventive purposes. The existence of such a specialty underscores the interest of Egyptian physicians in colorectal disease, further evidence of which is supplied by a papyrus entirely devoted to this pathology, Chester Beatty VI.[24] Elsewhere there is mention of "physicians of the belly" *(swnw shet*) who specialized in maladies of the uterus as well (the word *shet* having this double meaning in the popular language).[25]

A further type of specialist was associated with the epithet "one who knows the organs of the human body that are hidden from sight"—that is, a specialist in internal organs and what Herodotus (2.84) called "uncertain diseases." Jonckheere argued that he is better thought of as a consultant "whose advice was sought in connection with conditions that were difficult to diagnose or to treat, in the face of which the ordinary practitioner remained perplexed." The names of two physicians who practiced this specialty have come down to us, one of whom, Iry, is said to have known "the liquids dissolved in the humors."[26]

A final specialty is perhaps the most surprising of all. We know of it from a reference to Irenakhty, successor to Khuy at the court of Pepy I, who had been decorated with the title "interpreter of the liquids in the *netnetet*." This term designates a membrane or an organ having the form of a sac, perhaps the bladder. In that case Irenakhty may have been an expert in urinary disorders.[27]

What does this evidence of medical specialization tell us? It is difficult to draw any firm conclusions from the incomplete information that has survived: we know mainly names of physicians in the earlier periods; those of the New Kingdom and the Late Period remain largely unknown to us, the result of the development of magic, perhaps, and of the paucity of monuments bearing medical information that have been preserved from these times. We have records of 150 *swnww* for all of the epochs of pharaonic Egypt according to Boulu, even fewer according to Jonckheere (who reports 42 physicians for the Old Kingdom, 16 for the Middle Kingdom, 29 for the New Kingdom, and 11 for the Late Period). Boulu has discovered only 21 bearers of specialized titles, among whom oculists and dentists figure most prominently, owing to the recurrence of certain diseases in epigraphic accounts.[28]

Is this to say that the majority of Egyptian physicians did not practice as specialists? Or must we join Paul Ghalioungui in supposing that funerary inscriptions did not always mention physicians' specialties? On this view specialization existed very early in Egypt, in keeping with the tendency of primitive medicine there and elsewhere to consider each organ as an independent entity. Only later did the unity of the human body develop as a definite concept, accompanied by novel theories of

This limestone stele from Thebes (760–525 B.C.) shows a father and son, under a winged disk representing the sun, worshipping the mummiform figures of Osiris and Ra. The hieroglyphic text names the owner of the stele, a physician of the Third Intermediate or Late Period named Iretsekheru (also Irhorsekheru). Museum of Fine Arts, Boston.

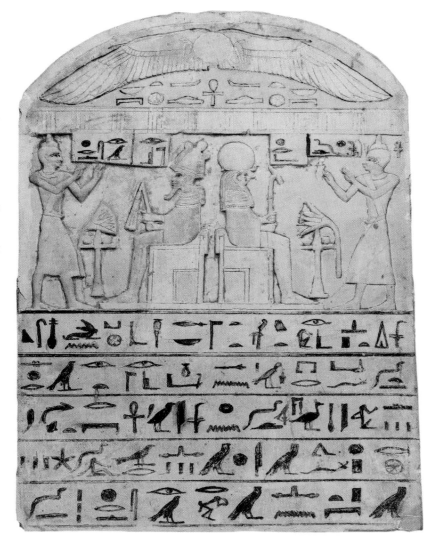

morbid humors. But this hypothesis does not explain the reappearance, confirmed by Herodotus, of specialist titles in the Late Period. And, as Ange Pierre Leca has objected, the assumption that medical art had advanced in the interval "contradicts the fixed character of Egyptian medicine through the centuries, which, so far from progressing, seems on the contrary to have deteriorated."[29]

Another possibility, proposed by Gérard Godron, is that Egyptian physicians were trained in a single specialty at the beginning of their careers and over time acquired additional knowledge, finally becoming full-fledged doctors. This would imply, by contrast with the system we know today, that the specialist occupied a lower social rank than the generalist *swnw*. In the final analysis, however, the simultaneous practice of several quite distinct specialties (as in the case of Khuy and Irenakhty) seems to point in another direction. Medical titles probably served more to inform patients about the extent of a physician's education, rather like the qualifications that general practitioners today often advertise, than to specify areas of actual concentration.[30]

Rights and Duties of the Profession

Egyptian society depended on the king, who, assisted by his top officials, oversaw civil and military administration. The medical profession in ancient Egypt was not an exception to the elaborate hierarchical structure that regulated the machinery of government, as the rich variety of titles and qualifications attached to physicians on funerary stelae and tomb inscriptions indicates.[31]

Thierry Bardinet has shown that the generic term *swnw* refers to low-ranking practitioners who had not managed to advance in grade. They were subject to the authority of an inspector of physicians (*sehedj swnw*), himself under the direction of a chief physician (*wer swnw*), whose mandate probably extended over a sizable geographical area. Appointed by the king, this powerful figure was responsible for looking after the health of his sovereign.[32]

Moreover, the royal palace, which under the Old Kingdom housed a great many departments, was the principal center of medical activities.[33] A medical corps in the exclusive service of the court was charged with the care not only of the king and his family but also of courtesans and a galaxy of servants. These court physicians, who were recruited from the most brilliant scholars outside the palace and who were considered to be the best practitioners in the kingdom, were themselves members of a strict hierarchy.[34] The lowest-ranking practitioners were answerable to an inspector and an overseer of palace physicians. At the top of the ladder was the king's personal doctor, the de facto chief physician of the north and the south *(wer swnw mehw shena),* who held authority over all practitioners, including those who lived outside the palace.[35] Even so, titles used outside did not necessarily have equivalents at court, and physicians who were eminent in civil practice were not necessarily integrated into the palace system at the same rank. But it was possible for everyone to gradually move up through the hierarchy, as the titles engraved on funerary monuments attest. We know, for example, that Iry, Nesemnaw, Nyankhra, and Khnumankh successively filled posts within the royal palace associated with the titles palace physician *(swnw per aa),* inspector of palace physicians *(sehedj swnw per aa),* and chief of palace physicians *(wer swnw per aa).*[36]

The court also included specialists equipped, as Bardinet has noted, with "particular knowledge in the domain of pathological causality."[37] Certain practitioners were competent in more than one specialty, such as Iry, styled royal oculist *(swnw irty per aa)* and royal physician of the belly *(swnw shet per aa),* and Khuy, chief dentist *(wer ibhy).*

This hierarchical regime was considerably modified during the Middle Kingdom: there were no longer inspectors of physicians, only physicians *(swnw)* subject to the authority of an overseer of physicians *(imy-r swnw)* and a chief physician *(wer swnw).*[38] In the New Kingdom, physicians to the king *(swnw n nesu)* constituted the base and the chief of physicians to the Lord of the Two Lands *(wer swnw n neb tawy)* was at the summit. We know the name of one of the latter, Iuti, who was chief physician to the Lord of the Two Lands and chief physician. It was only during the Late Period that palatine titles once again became frequent.[39]

Hierarchy and Secrecy

How did physicians move up through the various grades of the hierarchy? Perhaps with the approval of a supervisory body. Thus Gilles Boulu interprets two papyri, possibly from the temple of Amun at Karnak, that mention the existence of an "office (or department) of palace physicians."[40]

Such a body is mentioned in other writings as well. These documents attribute to it a regulatory function, notably with regard to the care given the king. One text, composed in the second year of the reign of Rameses IX by the king himself, instructs Ramesesnakht, the high priest of Amun, with regard to the high-quality ("twice good") galena that the pharaoh commanded to be sent for his eyedrops. The substance turned out to be unsatisfactory, as the text emphasizes: "When it was given to the physicians of the office of the physicians of the pharaoh [. . .] in order to treat [the condition], this galena was observed to be ineffective, having nothing in it that was worthy of being put into the eyedrops used by the pharaoh." It was returned with orders that a product of higher quality ("four times good") be sent in its place.[41]

A second, undated papyrus reproduces the text of a letter sent by a high dignitary, perhaps the vizier Neferrenpet, also of the Ramessid Period, to the chief doctor Thel:

> [X] speaks to the chief scribe and physician Thel of the temple of Amun and then to Ibhy [?] in these terms: I sent for you to prepare the twice-good galena in an elephant's tusk, [for] Pharaoh, my master said, "Make sure he brings it back again." When this letter reaches you, hasten to prepare this galena for Pharaoh and to send it along as quickly as possible. Understand that I have sent a letter to Hery, overseer of the domain of Amun and prophet of the temple of Khnum [?], regarding this matter. The divine father Wennefer of the temple of Amun will provide you with what you need. See that you are prudent, take care, and get under way.[42]

It is not known whether physicians were authorized to disclose the illnesses of their patients to third parties. Their medicines, it appears, did remain secret, for some medical knowledge seemed "jealously guarded by the physician." The theme of confidentiality is frequently encountered in the "Book of the Heart" of the Ebers papyrus (854–856), and occasionally in other places as well: "A secret treatment [drawn from the book] of plants that a physician customarily prepares" (Ebers 188). Some commentators have argued, however, that this notion of secrecy is wholly relative and would better be interpreted as referring to "that which is difficult to understand."[43]

Another aspect of medical confidentiality during the Greco-Roman period involved expert medical reports that physicians were called upon from time to time to furnish during trials for homicide or assault. But these later documents do not constitute a sufficient basis for asserting that this type of procedure existed in pharaonic Egypt proper.[44]

Were physicians paid as a function of their qualifications, their title, or their results? It is difficult to say, all the more so since money seems not to have appeared in ancient Egypt before the 30th Dynasty. Medical charges were settled in accordance with a barter system that was regulated for the most part by the state. Diodorus describes physicians as civil servants who were fed and housed by the government: "On their military campaigns and their journeys in the country [the Egyptians] all receive treatment without the payment of any private fee; for the physicians draw their support from public funds."[45]

Documents from Deir el-Medina throw some light on the nature of this subvention. The minimum monthly salary of doctors consisted of rations of cereal (wheat and barley), bread, and beer—in other words, the ingredients of a basic diet. An ostracon from the 20th Dynasty giving the scale of salaries paid to personnel at Deir el-Medina was initially supposed to show that physicians were the least well remunerated employees, since they received only one-quarter *khar* of one kind of grain (wheat) and one *khar* of another (barley) while ordinary workers received three and four *khars* respectively. But Jac Janssen has argued that the figure mentioned in fact represented a supplementary payment, above and beyond the basic wage received by workers. On this accounting, the total sum received by a physician would have approached that paid to the head of staff.[46] It is true that a passage in the Turin Canon, a papyrus dating from the New Kingdom, suggests that physicians were rather less well paid than scribes or porters: "Two *khar* of grain for two scribes, three *khar* for a porter, one *khar* for a physician." A fragment of the Vatican papyrus from the 19th Dynasty suggests, however, that physicians were also eligible to receive honoraria in the form of copper and natron, in addition to a monthly stipend, as in the case of a widower named Usihe who paid for services rendered to his late wife, Menatnofre.[47]

Remuneration was often proportional to the influence and reputation of the patient. Thus the physician Nebamun received from a Syrian prince and his wife slaves, cattle, copper, and natron. The pharaoh himself offered gold to some of his physicians and presented them with precious necklaces at official ceremonies, at least if we may trust the scene in the tomb chapel of Pentju, chief royal physician under Akhenaten, which shows him honored on three occasions with impressive necklaces made of gold in acknowledgment of his services. Palace physicians might also find themselves awarded, in addition to their usual salary, a burial chamber, furnishings for the afterlife, and a commemorative stele—gifts whose value was more symbolic than material.[48]

The majority of physicians, some of whom, according to Jonckheere, owned real estate and land, seem to have belonged to the middle class, along with priests, scribes, artisans, and certain skilled workers.[49] But physicians attached to the royal palace, like high officials, were undoubtedly elevated to the upper class.

2 Training and Practice

In trying to imagine what medical training was like in ancient Egypt, we must realize that the great majority of people did not have the benefit of a regular or structured education. It is estimated that in the Middle Kingdom, out of 1.5 million inhabitants, only between five and ten thousand adults knew how to read and write, which is to say between 0.33 and 0.66 percent of the population. In the New Kingdom, at Deir el-Medina, this proportion may have reached 5–7 percent or even higher.[1]

Methods of Instruction

Students of medicine underwent two kinds of training: individual instruction within the family and collective instruction given in schools. Education rested for the most part on the transmission of practical knowledge from one generation to another. Those who received an education subsequently became the sole providers for their entire families. According to Gustave Lefebvre, a physician personally communicated his learning to his sons, who, upon their father's death, inherited his privileges.[2] Diodorus Siculus observed in the first century B.C. that "the general mass of the Egyptians [. . .] are instructed from their childhood by their fathers or kinsmen in the practices proper to each manner of life," noting that "they are the only people where all the craftsmen are forbidden to follow any other occupation or belong to any other class of citizens than those stipulated by the laws and handed down to them from their parents." Evidence has been found of veritable medical dynasties, in particular that of the Iuny family during the New Kingdom.[3]

But apprentice physicians, like prospective priests and scribes, seem to have followed a course of general education as well, dispensed at the school of the palace or in the various "houses of life" *(per ankh)* in the land. Gilles Boulu has argued that this instruction lasted four years and ended at the age of ten, by which point pupils had learned to read and write correctly through the taking of dictation and recopying of texts, as the discovery of schoolboy notebooks suggests. Teaching was carried out in accordance with the harsh method of the paddle: "A boy's ear is on his back—he listens when he is hit."[4]

Once this phase of his training was finished, the future physician typically embarked upon an apprenticeship with his father or another close relative. Parents were not alone in taking responsibility for the child's education, as Georges Posener has noted:

> The tradition of paternal instruction was so well rooted in custom that all the didactic treatises are presented by their authors as advice given by father to son. Nonetheless kings entrusted princes and princesses of the blood to preceptors. Artisans and bureaucrats placed their offspring in apprenticeship. The next stage consisted in bringing several pupils together under the direction of a master. Group instruction was given at the court, where the high nobility sent their children to be educated together with the royal children. The various departments of government maintained centers for training, as did the temples.[5]

Sir Alan Gardiner was the first to propose that physicians completed their training in the houses of life. These centers, though they were physically part of the temples, constituted a distinct institution. In addition to other strictly theological activity, they contained departments devoted to magic and medicine in which "scribes of the house of life" (*hierogrammateis*, as they were called by the Greeks, which is to say literate men or scholars) tirelessly wrote down or recopied ancient religious and medical texts.[6] These men composed a "college of scholars," in Aksel Volten's phrase, "responsible for the protection of the life of the king and of the gods." It may be that the ancient texts dictated in these places were later reproduced in the medical papyri—manuals belonging to physicians that had been augmented by the commentaries of the most experienced scribes.[7]

The houses of life have also been compared to "centers of culture" in which scribes worked alongside professors, physicians, and astronomer-horologists. According to Lefebvre, they were supervised by elders who drew upon a body of empirical knowledge, particularly in connection with theology and medicine. The "master of the secrets of the house of life" and the "overseer of writings in the house of life" studied by Gardiner may have been just such figures.[8]

As for the existence of a medical department in these places, Boulu claims to have found proof in the biographical inscription adorning the statue of a certain Udjahorresnet, chief physician and chancellor under the pharaohs Ahmose II and Psamtek III.[9] Following the Persian invasion of the country in 525 B.C., Udjahorresnet was named chief of physicians by Cambyses while retaining his former title of chancellor. Summoned to the court at Susa, he remained a trusted advisor of Cambyses's successor, Darius I. To "ease people's minds"—the minds of the Egyptian people under Persian occupation—Darius instructed him to revive "schools of Egyptian thought":

> The Majesty of the King of Lower and Upper Egypt, Darius, may he
> live forever, commanded me to return to Egypt—while His Majesty
> was in Elam, when He was the great king of all foreign countries and
> grand sovereign of Egypt—to restore the buildings of the House of Life
> [devoted to] medicine, after they [had fallen into] ruin. The Barbarians
> carried me from country to country and brought me to Egypt, as the
> Lord of the Two Lands had ordered. I did as His Majesty had com
> manded me. I provided them with all their students, who were sons of
> persons of quality, there being no sons of ordinary people [there].[10]

If this inscription is to be believed, admission to the houses of life was granted on the basis of criteria that indicate, at least during the First Persian Period, some degree of social segregation. During the 26th Dynasty another chief of physicians, Peftjawaneith, appears to have been charged by the pharaoh Apries with restoring the houses of life in the temple of Osiris at Abydos.[11]

The major medical papyri that have come down to us suggest that the *wab*-priests of Sekhmet gave their apprentices theoretical instruction in the form of oral commentary on medical texts. By contrast, there is no clear evidence of clinical instruction involving patients in the houses of life. The only evidence we have, as Boulu has pointed out, comes from

Udjahorresnet himself, who claimed to have equipped his students with "all the necessary things indicated by the writings."[12]

An interesting piece of information about this institution is furnished by the physician Iuny's title: "He who knows the secrets of the chest of Bubastis." This chest appears to have contained surgical and other medical instruments. Additionally, the Cairo papyrus (no. 58,027) mentions the title "guardian of the myrrh of the house of life," which Frans Jonckheere has argued proves the existence of a "pharmaceutical department, attached to the medical department, in which medicines were prepared."[13]

Medical Practice

Egyptian physicians, like physicians today, conducted a clinical examination of their patients. And, like modern practitioners, they gave a diagnosis and established a prognosis in order to prescribe appropriate treatment. Thanks to the medical papyri, chiefly Ebers and Edwin Smith, it is possible to form some idea of the way the examinations were conducted.

Medical consultation, which Lefebvre has described as deliberate and solemn, consisted of three stages: examination, diagnosis, and prognosis. Examination began with a round of thorough questioning, in which the patient stated his complaints, that oriented the diagnosis toward a particular part of the anatomy: "If you question him about the affected place that is on him. . . ."[14] This also made it possible to evaluate the state of mind of the injured or sick person. In the Ebers papyrus (855z) we find this remark: "His inside *(ib)* is forgetful like someone who is thinking about something else."[15]

There followed an inspection of the face, urine, excrement, and expectoration. The practitioner meticulously examined wounds and deformations of the skin for signs of edema or hematoma and noted any trembling or symptoms of paralysis. No anomaly was neglected. In the case of injury to the bones or segments of the upper spinal column, for example, stiffness was observed: "His neck is heavy; it is not possible for him to look at his body" (Ebers 295).

For this purpose everything was useful. From the medical papyri we know that doctors relied not only on their sense of smell (in the second paragraph of the Kahun medical papyrus, for example, a gynecological ailment is described as having an odor of "burned meat") but also on the sense of touch. Palpation made it possible both to detect an abnormal fever and to search for abdominal tumors and wounds. In the course of examining the soft tissues for indications of an underlying osseous lesion, for example, the practitioner was able to feel crepitations—a sign of fracture (Edwin Smith 24). But palpation had above all a symbolic importance, enabling the physician to place himself in close contact with the patient by means of his fingers. This laying on of the hands, apart from its reassuring aspect, was intended to circumscribe illness and in some cases to extirpate it.

It is unclear whether Egyptian physicians manually checked the patient's pulse or, if they did, whether they knew what it signified. The gloss of a phrase found in the Edwin Smith papyrus—"As for 'when you examine a man,' it means counting things with a bushel [that is, a measure of wheat] or counting something with the fingers"—has given rise to various interpretations. J. G. W. Gispen, Bendix Ebbell, and James Henry Breasted all affirmed the existence of this practice.[16] In their view, Egyptian medicine was a major influence on the Greek anatomist and surgeon Herophilus (ca. 330–260 B.C.), traditionally regarded as the first to have recognized the importance of the pulse, which he measured by means of a clepsydra (or water clock). Egyptian physicians themselves made use of such a clock as early as the 18th Dynasty under Thutmose III, and excavations at Giza have uncovered an example from the time of Merenptah during the 19th Dynasty.[17] For the moment, however, the question remains undecided. But even if physicians did not count the pulse it is reasonable to suppose, as Dominique Spaeth has argued, that they "examined [it] qualitatively (in terms of strength and rhythm) and semi-quantitatively (slow or accelerated), though the writings so far discovered do not mention this." Moreover, the medical papyri do seem to indicate that the importance of repeated examinations in monitoring a patient's recovery from illness was well understood.[18]

Following this rigorous and rational examination, carried out in accordance with a set procedure, the physician went on to state the various symptoms and functional signs (all forty-eight cases of the Edwin Smith papyrus begin with the phrase "If you examine a man having . . ."). He then pronounced both a diagnosis ("You will say what is the matter with him: a patient who suffers from . . .") and a prognosis indicating the seriousness of the case. While the variability of prognoses suggests that physicians knew their limitations, it is clear too that they did not abandon the incurably ill, but instead cared for them.

The rational aspects of medical practice, based upon thorough clinical examination, must not be allowed to obscure the essentially pragmatic nature of Egyptian medicine. The Egyptians were interested above all in symptoms, such as cough and fever, and only occasionally were they able to identify an actual syndrome. This concentration on surface signs of illness was nonetheless part of an original approach to nosology that conceived of diseases as entities in their own right, worthy of being combated. Physicians treated patients with medicine and magic, separately or in combination, in order to make treatment as effective as possible by "acting upon the mind" of the sick person and, not incidentally, by "acting in such a way that the privileges associated with the exercise of a particularly profitable profession would continue to be reserved for an elite." Not only did Egyptian physicians understand the importance of mental states in struggling against disease four thousand years before Freud; their social position gave them additional incentive to resort to magic when medical remedies proved insufficient.[19]

But it should not be supposed that physicians were free to treat the patient as they pleased. To the contrary, they had to respect the ancient texts of their profession with the greatest scrupulousness. These writings, because they were considered products of divine inspiration, were held to be sacred and therefore immutable. We have the testimony of Diodorus, who emphasized that Egyptian physicians

> administer their treatments in accordance with a written law which was composed in ancient times by many famous physicians. If they follow the rules of this law as they read them in the sacred book and yet are unable to save their patient, they are absolved from any charge and go unpunished; but if they go contrary to the law's prescriptions in any respect, they must submit to a trial with death as the penalty, the lawgiver holding that but few physicians would ever show themselves wiser than the mode of treatment which had been closely followed for a long period and had been originally prescribed by the ablest practitioners.

Aristotle, who lived at the time of the last native-born pharaohs, indicated moreover that in Egypt, physicians had "the right to alter their prescription after four days, although if one of them alters it before [then] he does so at his own risk."[20]

The Egyptians were the first to formulate norms of therapeutic procedure—a particularly fruitful advance in the history of medical thought. Nonetheless it may be wondered whether habitual deference to ancient teachings and blind respect for tradition did not in fact limit the progress of pharaonic medicine.

Physicians and Magicians

The therapeutic use of magic by the Egyptians reflected a conception of the world in which, as Gonzague Bontemps puts it, "everything was significant and chance did not exist." Regulating this use of magic were four fundamental concepts, admirably described by Paul Ghalioungui. According to the first, the principle of identity, the representation of an individual plant, organ, or symptom—the utterance or writing of its name—was sufficiently powerful to enable it to be acted upon. Medicinal properties could be inferred on the basis of a correspondence with appearance or sound as well. A red stone, for example, was thought to stop bleeding.[21]

The second principle, of solidarity, associated all the parts of the body with one another. Thus the Egyptians thought it was possible to act on an individual patient by means of a lock of hair or even a scrap of clothing. The third principle, of homeopathy, posited that "like evokes like," which is to say that "two events that follow one another once will necessarily follow one another in the future." The fourth and final principle, inspired by the legend of Isis and Osiris, linked death with the image of "a protracted sleep."[22]

Magical medicine rested above all upon speech: corresponding to each condition were formulas to be recited. A manual ritual might be associated with a particular condition as well, along with objects that were to be handled in certain ways. The aim was to deflect the curses that magic, a dangerous technique, was liable to bring upon the practitioner. Thus one finds at the outset of the Ebers papyrus three paragraphs meant to protect the physician who relied on its guidance. As Bardinet has emphasized, these paragraphs serve as a kind of "magical prologue" to the body of the papyrus.[23]

The first two sections immunized the physician against the potential

People of all classes wore amulets to protect health and ensure well-being both in this life and in the hereafter. Many amulets were shaped like living creatures, or parts of them, in the belief that the wearer could assimilate their desirable characteristics. An amulet's symbolism and purpose were associated not only with its shape but also with the material from which it was made. From top left to bottom right: *djed*-pillar, *wedjat*-eye, papyrus bud, and crocodile (all of faience); square (obsidian); Horus falcon (faience); heart shape (stone); head of the god Bes (faience). Aegyptisches Museum, Berlin.

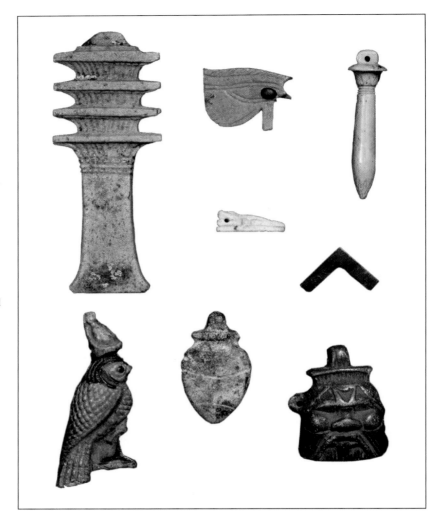

dangers of contact with the patient and his environment of vindictive demons. In these texts the divine origin of the formulas is established, and physicians and magicians are said to imitate Thoth, the benevolent god charged by Ra with the protection of a "suffering humanity," who had transmitted his science and power to them. Thus the Ebers papyrus opens with these lines:

I have come from Heliopolis in the company of the great ones of the temples, the guarantors of protection, the sovereigns of eternity. I have also come from Sais, in the company of the mother of the gods. They have given me their protection. [Thus] I possess the utterances that the lord of the universe has devised to drive out the doings of a god, a goddess, a dead man, a dead woman, and so on, that are in this my head, in this my neck, in these my shoulders, in this my flesh, in these my limbs, and [I have the utterances] to punish the Slanderer, the leader of those who cause disorder to enter into this my flesh by gnawing at these my bodily parts, by entering into this very flesh, into this my head, into these my shoulders, into this my skin, into these my bodily parts. I belong to the god Ra. He has said: It is I who will protect him against his enemies. Thoth is his guide, he who has made it happen that I speak writing, who has caused medical complications, and given the power to the learned men and physicians who are in his retinue to relieve [the sick]. I am the one who is beloved of the god, he keeps me alive. Words to be recited when placing a medication on any suffering place of the body of a man. Truly effective, a million times.

The third paragraph offers guidance for the physician who has nonetheless fallen ill, a victim of retaliation by the demons against whom he struggles every day.

Following this prologue, the verbal part of the ritual continues with incantations. Their efficaciousness resided in the form, the sound, and the rhythm of the words spoken, and rested upon a fourfold principle of transfer, artificial myths, incomprehensible formulas, and magical impressions. The first aspect, transfer, consisted in displacing the condition experienced by the patient into the divine world. Chester Beatty V, 4, gives an example of a protective text intended to treat migraine, symbolized here by serpents: "Spell for driving out migraine. The head of such a one, male or female, is the head of Osiris Wennefer, on whose head were placed 367 divine serpents, which spit flames, to force them to let go of the head of such a [male], son of such a [female], like the head of Osiris."[24] Through this incantation the doctor-magician gave a rational explanation for the affliction by transferring it to the divine world. For the gods, healing the patient was the only way to restore order to the world.

A second element of treatment involved the invention of ad hoc myths, since traditional mythology did not contain a divine analogue for every one of the many woes known to human beings.[25] Thus some incantations, such as one in the Hearst papyrus (214), refer to Horus as having sustained both a snake's bite and a scorpion's sting as well as a wound to the head.

In addition to previously unknown myths, the doctor-magician exploited the very obscurity of his own utterances, which impressed the patient much more forcefully than a clear formula. In the glosses of the London medical papyrus, for example, one finds many words in various foreign languages: "Warding off of the Canaanite malady according to what the inhabitants of Keftiu [Crete] say about it: [O] senti, [O] kapupi, far from [me], O Yamentiro, [O] karo. May this formula be pronounced upon: fermented liquid *(gachu)*, urine; *sedjet*. To be applied to it" (London 2).

A final aspect of magical technique concerned not the living but the dead. Doctor-magicians who failed to save their patients had to redeem themselves by protecting the deceased during passage to the afterlife. Some of them made use of figurines meant to ward off the "dangerous dead," mutilating or spiking the hieroglyphics representing harmful animals with knives. Thus the character of the lion is sometimes found cut in two in the Old Kingdom; in the Middle Kingdom the snake is subjected to the same treatment or else is decapitated.[26]

Priestly Therapeutics   Magical techniques were not the only link between medicine and religion. Medicine was also practiced in sanatoriums inside the temples, where patients came to experience therapeutic dreams.

Sick persons in search of cures began to visit these places in the Late Period and frequented them throughout the Ptolemaic era. Two in particular, in the "Holy of Holies" temple in Deir el-Bahri and the temple of Hathor at Dendera, are known to us from surviving descriptions. The first was hollowed out of a mountain on the west bank of the Nile, across from Thebes, on the order of Queen Hatshepsut. Its upper terrace was dedicated to Imhotep and Amenhotep during the Ptolemaic era. The sick were welcomed in the outermost of the temple's two chapels: there a deep voice suddenly came out of the darkness, announcing the indicated cure. In this way sick persons were persuaded that supernatural intervention would assist their recovery. Graffiti such as this one have been found on the walls of the shrine, probably engraved or painted by patients waiting to be cured: "Andromachus, a Macedonian, a laborer, came to the good god Amenhotep; he was sick and the god cured him the same day."[27]

The temple at Dendera, consecrated to the god Hathor, housed an extensive hydrotherapy center approached by a corridor of healing statues. Streams fed stone tanks of different sizes in which the sick bathed in the hope of being cured. In both this temple and the one at Deir el-Bahri, therapeutic dreams were induced as well, during the one or more nights that patients spent in the sanatorium after witnessing an entire day of ceremony. Since sleep was considered the means by which one was transported to the kingdom of the dead, the sick were able to question the gods and plead to be restored to health.[28]

Medicines and Pharmacists

The Egyptian pharmacopoeia was exceptionally rich. It is perhaps the source of modern pharmaceutics, if only etymologically. Riad has suggested that the Greek term *pharmakon* comes from the Egyptian *peh-ir-maki,* meaning "he who brings security"—one of the characterizations of Thoth, the celebrated ibis-headed god of scribes who was associated with healing.[29] Medicinal preparations were often long, complicated, and above all very numerous, as though Egyptian practitioners hoped by multiplying them to achieve the greatest possible effectiveness, fortified still further by the recitation of magical formulas. We should nonetheless be cautious in assigning an exact interpretation to these remedies, for many of the ingredients that figure in the recipes for them, such as "eye of the sky," "costly ointment," "tail of rat," "head of donkey," and "tooth of hog," remain unknown to us—and this despite the 240 translations proposed by Ebbell for some 400 names of drugs mentioned in the Ebers papyrus. To these one may add 358 accepted translations, 167 doubtful or unrecognized ones, and 19 illegible hieroglyphs contained in Hermann Grapow's study of some 500 pharmacological ingredients.

Even if we are not sure of all of these ingredients, we do know that the medicines mentioned in the medical papyri were prepared in accordance with precise, clear, well-organized instructions. First came a statement and numbering of the various substances used together with the

The dwarf god Bes was the protector of children. An ailing child might be fed from a Bes-shaped bottle like this one in the hope that the god would cure its illness. If this remedy was not effective, a physician would be summoned. The bottle shown here, made of iron oxide pigment, ceramic, and human hair, dates from the Late Period (664–332 B.C.). Rosicrucian Egyptian Museum, San Jose, California.

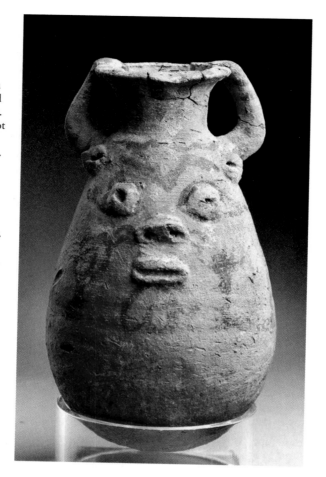

proportions (since ingredients were measured by volume rather than by weight) to be observed. The chief unit of measure was the bushel *(heqat),* equivalent to roughly 4.5 liters (about 4.75 quarts), initially provided for cereals and, in the most detailed recipes, given in fractions.[30] Quantities of ingredients, either individually or added together, or sometimes the size of a total dose of medicine to be administered, were frequently expressed in terms of the *henu,* equal to 1/10 of a *heqat* or about 450 milliliters (a little less than half a quart). The smallest volume measure, nearly equivalent to our tablespoon, about 14 milliliters, was the *ro* (1/320 of a *heqat*).[31] Accompanying this list of ingredients were technical instructions for making the medicine in question, whether by crushing, cooking, mixing, or some other method. Beer, wine, water, and honey furnished the most common vehicles for ingesting the active substance.

Instructions were given, finally, regarding the manner in which remedies were to be administered. The Egyptians used potions, gargles and mouthwashes, herbal teas, various decoctions and steepings, pills, lozenges, pellets, poultices, ointments, ophthalmic and auricular salves, plasters, eyedrops, inhalations, fumigations, suppositories, enemas, tampons, and vaginal injections. To this long list may be added pastes that were applied to decayed teeth or smeared on a wet nurse's breasts before feeding. It is interesting that recipes often specify the age of the patients in question, the hour when the medicine is to be taken, the day, the season, and the duration of the treatment. Sometimes even the temperature of a preparation is indicated: "[It] is to be heated and taken at a temperature agreeable to the finger" (Ebers 799).

The Egyptian pharmacy rested essentially on three types of substances—mineral, vegetable, and animal—having therapeutic properties.[32] Thus alabaster was used in the preparation of ointments for the skin (Ebers 714–715, Hearst 153–154), and yellow ochre (a clay rich in hydrated iron oxide) to treat trachoma and alopecia. Galena (lead sulfide) and pinchbeck (an alloy of copper and zinc) occur in ophthalmological recipes. A host of other mineral substances were used for similar therapeutic purposes: arsenic sulfide, brick and earthenware made from clay, soil, granite, gypsum, "Memphis stone" (no doubt limestone), malachite, millstone chips, mud, sand, soot, and antimony.

Plants were a source of laxatives (the fruit of the sycamore, colocynth, figs, the ricinus or castor-oil plant, and aloe) as well as diuretics (juniper berries, bryum, and spring squill). Brewer's yeast, recommended by the ancient Egyptians for the treatment of intestinal infections and skin diseases, contains vitamin B and possesses antibiotic properties against staphylococcus.

Animal and human substances entered into the composition of more than half of the 1,740 recorded recipes that have come down to us. Apart from honey, frequently mentioned for its soothing, antibacterial, and antifungal properties, the Egyptians favored cow's milk, animal fats and fresh meat (particularly liver, rich in vitamin A, as an ophthalmological remedy). There is abundant evidence that what might be called excremental therapy, which made use of droppings, urine, flyspecks, and so on, was commonly employed as well. Today this surprising form of treatment is the object of much scholarly curiosity.[33]

The medical papyri suggest that physicians were personally responsible for preparing these recipes. But they may have had help from assistants with whom they shared their secrets. A worksite attendance record, inscribed on an ostracon from the New Kingdom, reveals that the worker Paherypedjet acted as a dispenser of medicines for several persons—a responsibility that might be described by several titles. More generally, pharmaceutical preparation may have been the responsibility of a department, perhaps within houses of life, whose head bore the title "administrator of those who make medicines" *(kherep mesyuhem).*[34] We know that plants, which had once been the province of a *sem*-priest (also known as the "medicinal plant man"), were stored in these places under the supervision of a "guardian of the myrrh of the house of life."[35] It seems likely that these men were the remote ancestors of modern-day pharmacists.

Surgical Instruments Despite the remarkable precision of the surgical observations in the Edwin Smith papyrus, the instruments and methods employed are not clearly described. Indeed, they are mentioned only in passing in the paragraphs devoted to various treatments. The meager information we have has nonetheless been fleshed out by the results of archaeological excavations, which have brought to light a range of probable surgical instruments that constitute direct evidence of the surpassing technological skill of the Egyptians.[36]

Among these items one finds three kinds of knife (*des, ses,* and *nepet*), forceps *(hemehu),* even rush stems, which were used solely to make incisions. But it is very difficult to place these relics in any precise correspondence with modern instruments. A great many items have come down to us that, for lack of a better term, can only be characterized as "surgical" in nature. Embalming tools, however, have been perfectly preserved and identified: straight scalpels, lancets, knives with a blade that is rounded at the tip and the base, and copper and bronze knives.

Also identified have been sharpened stones used in circumcision, as well as straight and curved forceps. A number of these instruments are depicted in the Roman Period temple of Kom Ombo.[37]

One instrument, a kind of tapered and sharpened blade that was probably used to puncture and probe tumefactions, is of particular interest. Having first been heated over fire, the blade would have facilitated the removal of tumors and abscesses by cauterizing the wound. In this connection two types of cautery were distinguished: the *hemem* (Ebers 872), probably a metallic cautery or fire-heated lancet; and the *dja,* or "firestick" (Edwin Smith 39), whose hieroglyph appears in texts from the earliest dynasties. The latter tool was a sort of drill whose sharpened tip was placed in a cavity dug into a block of wood. When it was rotated between open hands, or with the use of a bow, a spark shot up, lighting the pointed end of the stick. This rudimentary device made it possible to cauterize abscesses, boils, and the like.

The ingenuity of Egyptian practitioners was remarkable. Thus, for example, the Edwin Smith papyrus tells us that a case of cephalic tetanus was treated by means of a reed through which a cooling drink or liquid nourishment was introduced into the patient's mouth. The Ebers papyrus mentions an identical reed, only beveled, used to pierce and drain a fluid-filled tumor. Eye doctors also used a long and flexible reed (or else the quill of a vulture feather) to inject drops into a diseased eye.

Bandaging

For the dressing of wounds the Egyptians preferred linen to wool, which was considered impure. Cotton had not yet appeared in Egypt and was not known to them. Flax (originally *Linum humile,* now classified as *Linum usitatissimum*) had been cultivated in Egypt from very early times, however, and linen had been made from it since the Neolithic period, in predynastic and dynastic eras alike. The Egyptians made use of linen in treating wounds and in the form of bandages as a support for dressings.[38]

In direct contact with wounds they put compresses made of shredded linen, or linen swabs, which had the property of absorbing serous fluids. These strips of cloth were also used to provide support for pharmacological preparations, typically consisting of fat and honey.[39] One thinks of the prescription for snakebite, a moist compress containing desert sand, mentioned in the Brooklyn papyrus (44); also the piece of dry

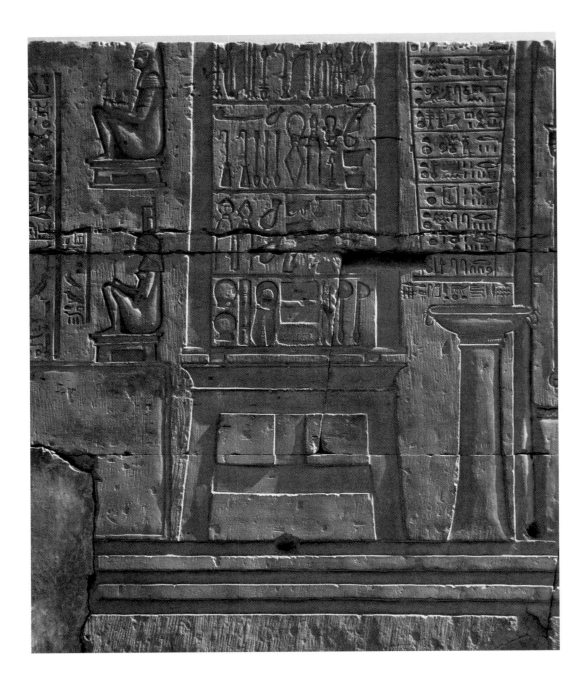

lint, referred to in the Edwin Smith papyrus (28), that was placed at the opening of a neck wound penetrating as far as the trachea.[40] In Breasted's view, this patch may have been meant to drain the pus by capillarity, in place of the traditional dressing of honey and fat.[41]

Fresh meat, whose astringent and homeostatic character imparted a soothing effect, was most often recommended as a dressing for open wounds on the first day, followed by a preparation of honey, fat, and plant fiber until the wound had finally healed.[42] The Hearst papyrus also calls for the immediate application of raw meat to crocodile bites— a treatment that had its origin in the ancient belief that the meat of a recently slaughtered animal was still suffused with life.

Honey, for its part, possesses hygroscopic properties that give it an antiseptic effect by modifying the environment in which germs develop, thus offering partial protection against the infection of wounds. But sweet substances in general were known empirically to promote the healing of wounds and ulcers.

Fat was converted by heating into a soap valued for its soothing quality, and also for preventing linen swabs from sticking to wounds. Beeswax was sometimes used in these recipes too, along with parts of various trees and plants: locust *(Acacia vera)* and willow, recommended for their astringent action; sycamore and jujube, known for their effectiveness against snake venom; also carob, mallow, melilot, the castor-oil plant, valerian, and onion.

A variety of minerals and liquids were locally applied as well. Minerals included alum, minium (cinnabar or red lead), "salt of the north" (natron), copper filings, and red ochre. Milk, oil, wine, and water often served as excipients to give medicinal preparations the desired volume or consistency. The soothing properties of fermented products such as beer, barley gum, dates, and flour were also recognized.

Linen bandages came in various sizes. Their tight weave helped protect wounds against infection by holding dressings in place while at the

The implements depicted in the middle panel of this frieze in the Roman Period temple at Kom Ombo strongly resemble tools used by surgeons today, including forceps and scalpels. At left are two women in labor, seated on low birthing stools; at right is a washbasin. From the wall of the outer corridor, temple of Sobek and Horus (third century B.C.).

same time providing a high degree of mechanical stability in the case of gaping wounds and fractures. Breasted expressed great admiration for the extraordinary technique displayed by Egyptian embalmers in applying and arranging bandages as part of the process of mummification. From there it is but a small step to suppose that Egyptian physicians had acquired equal competence in using bandages to bind up wounds, as Jonckheere has done, pointing to descriptions of a series of crisscrossed ("figure eight") wrappings for the head, simple spicas for the groin and the pelvis, dolabriform ("axhead") coverings for the limbs, and overlapping rolls for the feet.[43]

This same linen fabric, cut into strips, was used to hold splints in place in order to immobilize fractures (Edwin Smith 37). Lefebvre believes the splints were covered with cloth before being applied—a form of padding observed in the case of a fourteen-year-old girl whose broken right thighbone was held in place by four wooden splints, covered with linen and attached to the thigh as far down as the knee; and in that of a man whose fractured forearm was stabilized by three splints made of bark covering the elbow and the wrist. Reserved for an entirely different use, though made from the same material, were delicate bandages called *awi* or *aawi,* always mentioned in pairs in connection with the treatment of wounds. These were applied as an adhesive plaster across a gaping wound, drawing together the lips of the wound to accelerate healing.[44]

Other substances that may have been used as adhesives, or have been incorporated into such materials, include beeswax (whose cultivation went back to the Old Kingdom, as certain bas-reliefs attest) and *diapalme,* or palm wax.[45] Wax is mentioned in several pharmacological preparations in the Brooklyn papyrus, though its type has not been identified. The Egyptians also manufactured a glue from animal by-products (bone, skin, cartilage, and tendons, ground up into a gelatinous mass that was boiled and then dried by evaporation), as well as gum resins derived from bdellium, myrrh, and various species of the acacia tree found in Egypt and the Sudan. Resins extracted mainly from certain conifers of the eastern region of the Mediterranean basin, such as the cedar of Lebanon, the Cilician fir, and the Aleppo pine, also served as adhesive material.

But what was done when a wound needed to be completely closed? The Edwin Smith papyrus (47) indicates that the Egyptians sutured gaping wounds with thread. According to Lefebvre, the threads used for this purpose came from the intestine of an animal, cut up into thin strips. Sir W. M. Flinders Petrie believed he had found needles that could have been used for this kind of procedure.[46]

Antiseptics and Analgesics
The Egyptians were also familiar with substances having antiseptic effects. One recipe in the Edwin Smith papyrus (41), no doubt the product of long experience, calls for a decoction of willow leaves to be applied to an infected wound to the chest. Willow bark, from which salicin is extracted, is also known to possess astringent and antipyretic properties. Other vegetable substances, such as barley flour, also acted as anti-inflammatory agents, as did a vasodilatory preparation applied to snakebites, mentioned in the Brooklyn papyrus, consisting of jujube ash mixed with vinegar and onion.

Then there is a curious substance called *imrw*, mentioned seven times in the Edwin Smith treatise, whose medicinal use in the Roman Period was noted by Pliny. Other Egyptian texts refer to it as an astringent. Breasted thought it served to disinfect unclean wounds, and guessed that it was alum, a mineral extracted at the mines of Dakhla and Kharga in the desert west of the Nile Valley.[47] Other useful minerals included copper, scraps of which were applied to snakebites (Brooklyn 51c) to alleviate the virulence of the venom. Copper oxide, noted for its resolvent and astringent action, was mixed with zinc oxide to yield an ointment employed in the treatment of boils and carbuncles.

There is some evidence that the Egyptians knew how to relieve pain by means of anesthetics of one kind or another. In addition to the opium poppy *(Papaver somniferum)* and mandrake, both represented on bas-reliefs and necklaces, researchers have been interested in the "magic stone"—limestone from the vicinity of Memphis. Dioscorides states that the Egyptians practiced a form of local anesthesia with this stone *("Memphites lithos"),* grinding it into a powder and applying it to the affected part of the body.[48] Pliny, for his part, described it as marble mixed with vinegar, which would have triggered the release of carbon dioxide. John Nunn points out, however, that while inhalation of carbon dioxide at concentrations of more than 20 percent may lead to loss of consciousness, it does not cause what strictly speaking would be called anesthesia. Louis Baslez, in his study of poisons in Egypt, suggested that it was either an asphalt, which, on contact with flame, released bituminous fumes in quantities large enough to daze the patient, or a siliceous stone coated with an opium-based narcotic.[49]

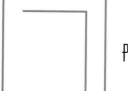

PART II

REVELATIONS OF PALEOPATHOLOGY

3 Mummification

The aim of paleopathology—the science of diseases whose existence can be demonstrated from human and animal remains—is to penetrate the mysteries of mummified corpses through the use of scientific methods, particularly in the domain of Egyptian medicine. Apart from the pathological and related information that can be obtained from their analysis, mummies have long been of interest to medicine because the distinctive character of Egyptian funerary ritual was believed to show that a sophisticated anatomical knowledge had been placed in the service of the treatment of disease. The first modern error has been to believe that the Egyptians' perfect mastery of the technique of mummification made them the fathers of modern anatomy. The second has been to suppose, following Pliny, that they commonly conducted autopsies with a scientific purpose in mind, namely, to determine the causes of death.[1]

Embalmers and Physicians

We know that the practice of autopsy was current during the Greco-Roman period in the school of Alexandria under the leadership of Erasistratus and Herophilus. But it is unlikely that Egyptian physicians of the pharaonic era, who identified cadavers with "the flesh of Osiris," ever undertook systematic dissections, for fear of committing a desecration.[2] This reluctance would explain the confusion that exists in the description of arteries, veins, and lymphatic and glandular ducts, all designated by the generic name of *metu*, meaning "canals" or "vessels."

Some authors have nonetheless supposed that Egyptian physicians, having witnessed the work of embalmers at first hand, drew upon their expertise. Gustave Lefebvre held that the ancient practice of embalming had made it possible for the Egyptians to establish, if not actually a body of knowledge, then at least a conception of anatomy unknown to other oriental peoples. Marc-Adrien Dollfus has argued that the observations of the Edwin Smith papyrus indicate that physicians were familiar with the work of embalmers through written accounts, if not also through personal experience.[3] Indeed, one case explicitly mentions a "Book of the Embalmer" (Edwin Smith 19).

Several families are known to have produced both doctors and embalmers. A donation stele at Abydos, from the Middle Kingdom, refers to a doctor named Nemtyemhat by the title "chief of physicians and of the *kherep* priests of *Serqet*," to his brother Kheduy as "priest *(sem)* and embalmer [of Anubis]," and to his son Tatu as both lector priest *(khery-hebet)* and "one with authority over the mysteries of the hall of embalming" *(hery-tep)*. The existence of these titles within a single family suggests that such a relationship was not accidental, and justifies the inference that its members enjoyed a common technical training.[4]

But even if some degree of contact between the two professions is probable, the balance of the evidence available to us suggests that the anatomical knowledge possessed by the physicians of ancient Egypt came mainly from examination of injured human subjects and from anatomical studies carried out on animals. It is significant that the hieroglyphic symbols for the heart, tongue, teeth, and uterus contain animal determinatives—proof that the homology of human and animal organs was recognized, a sign of the influence of comparative anatomy.

The Order of the World

The practice of mummification in ancient Egypt grew out of a fundamental conception of human nature. Man was considered to be not a unitary being, but rather a complex creature constituted by eight closely related elements. Four of these were physical in character: the body *(khet)*, which is to say the carnal shell, or mortal coil of the individual; the name; the heart; and the shadow. The other four were of a spiritual nature: the *akh*, the *ka*, the *ba*, and the *sahu*. Death dissociated the material components from the immaterial ones, the latter group living on outside the bodily cloak of the deceased person. It was therefore essential to preserve the body after death, eliminating all possibility of decomposition so that the *ka* and the *ba* would be capable of "recognizing" the physical shell that had been their host during life on earth, for the reintegration of these elements was the necessary condition of the *akh*'s rising up from the body to the divine tribunal.[5]

The purpose of mummification, then, was to create a suitable receptacle for the spiritual elements of the personality, which were indispensable to life in the hereafter. The symbolism of mortuary ritual was meant to persuade human beings that they helped to maintain the order of the world, both in life and in death, by establishing a bridge between earthly existence and the afterlife. The function of the pharaoh, for his part, was to guarantee and perpetuate this order, a responsibility that had been handed down to him by the gods.

Justification for the practice of mummification—"the passage between the two lives"—was found in the myth of Isis and Osiris. The legend of the Ennead related that Geb, god of the earth, and Nut, goddess of the sky, lived at the beginning of time and begot two sons, Osiris and Seth, and two daughters, Isis and Nephthys. Osiris married his sister Isis (also called "the great one of magic," according to an epigraphical text in the temple at Philae) and reigned with her on earth. Seth and Nephthys, who had also married each other, represented their exact antithesis. Seth, overcome by jealousy, resolved to do away with Osiris. He secretly had a superb chest built to his brother's measurements. Then, taking advantage of the opportunity offered by a banquet, he displayed the chest to the other guests and promised to make a gift of it to whoever could fit into it. When Osiris innocently climbed inside, Seth and his accomplices closed the lid and threw the chest, now transformed into a coffin, into the Nile.

Isis set out at once in search of her husband's body, traveling the length and breadth of the country, and soon learned that the chest had washed up on the shores of Byblos in Phoenicia, at the foot of a small tree. There she recovered Osiris's corpse and took it back to Egypt for burial. Furious at this, Seth cut Osiris's body into thirty-six pieces, which he then dispersed throughout the kingdom.

Isis, having managed at last to locate all these parts, embalmed them and reassembled them with the aid of bandages. She then assumed the guise of a sparrow hawk, lowered herself onto Osiris's phallus, and so conceived a son, Horus, who would grow up to overthrow Seth and take power. Meanwhile Osiris, mummified and deified, became the god of the underworld—"the divine archetype of the mummy who preserves the body for eternity," as Guy Rachet has put it. "The mummified body is identified with Osiris, in thus taking his name, which is added to the name borne by the living person."[6]

The Origins of Mummification

Thanks to the study of texts and of mummies themselves, this "act of faith," as it might well be called, sacralized and faithfully carried out according to rites that were recorded in writing and deeply rooted in religious tradition, is today perfectly understood, even if it took many years to work out the actual techniques of embalming.

The idea of mummifying the dead seems to have appeared first during the Predynastic Period, when bodies were buried in simple pit-graves dug in the desert. The Egyptians would have known from experience, having witnessed the havoc wreaked upon the contents of these primitive graves by wind and animals, the dessicating effects of the hot sand and the extremely dry climate, as well as the excellent state of preservation of the bodies exposed to them. The burning sand that enveloped mortal remains rapidly absorbed roughly 75 percent of the water they contained, largely arresting the process of decomposition. Under these conditions a body lost about three-quarters of its weight, and the skin hardened until it resembled leather. A desire to provide even more effective protection for the dead led to the building, from the time of the 1st Dynasty, of formal funerary structures known as *mastaba*-tombs. Coffins made of wickerwork or wood were placed in an underground brick-lined chamber, furnished with a chapel and all the objects the deceased person would need in the afterlife, but these measures were not enough to stem the normal processes of putrefaction. Deprived of the drying action of the sand, bodies preserved in the new tombs gradually decomposed, so that only their bones remained.[7]

Early Experiments

The first successful attempts at preserving cadavers occurred at the beginning of the Old Kingdom. During the first three dynasties, the body was placed in the fetal position, wrapped very tightly in linen bandages that had been soaked in resin to preserve its shape, and isolated from its immediate environment. Over time this method was refined, giving rise to the "false mummies" of the 3rd Dynasty: the corpse was dried out, until only skin was left on the bones, and the body was then reconstituted around the skeleton by means of a kind of stuffing, or padding, made from resin-soaked shreds of linen.[8]

By the early 4th Dynasty embalmers understood the role of putrefaction in causing the viscera to decompose. These organs were now removed from the abdomen by means of an incision made to the left side, thereby bringing about a definitive change from the fetal to the supine position. The viscera extracted from the body were preserved in canopic jars filled with a solution of natron (a natural carbonate of crystallized sodium extracted from the salt lakes found in the area of Wadi el-Natrun—whence the name—between Cairo and Alexandria), which completely absorbs the moisture of organs and tissues.[9] Toward the end of the 5th Dynasty, evisceration was accompanied by a more elaborate form of bandaging, covered by a layer of plaster or resin and meant to suggest the clothing worn by the deceased person. Facial features, molded with plaster, were painted as well. But even though bodies preserved their shape, decomposition continued to occur beneath the bandages, which in the end formed only an empty shell around the skeleton. The first concern of the embalmers, then, was to remove the body from every possible source of putrefaction, using natron after evisceration in order to ensure the drying out of body tissues.

It was also during this period that embalmers began to be recognized as a distinct corporate body, paid for their work by gifts in kind—typically reclaimed offerings to the gods—or otherwise by various remunerations furnished by the family of the deceased person. Despite these advantages they seem not to have enjoyed high social position. Mummification, which until the end of the Old Kingdom had been reserved for kings and eminent dignitaries, now became available in simplified form to the upper and middle classes, albeit with only qualified success. The first embalming instruments and materials known to us, often found buried in a small shaft not far from the tomb, date from the Middle Kingdom.[10]

Mummification in the New Kingdom

A decisive advance in the techniques of mummification, which made them both more labor-intensive and more effective, coincided with the advent of the 18th Dynasty, when they reached their highest degree of perfection, as the particularly well preserved royal mummies of the period attest.[11] The ritual of embalming was carried out in accordance

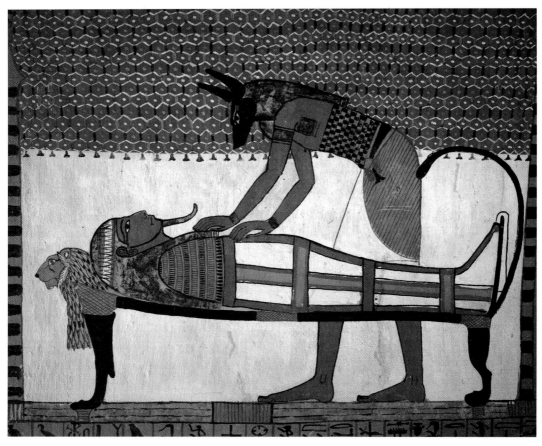

Anubis, god of the dead, is shown laying his hands upon the mummy of Sennutem, a necropolis official of the early Rammesid period. It is thought that embalmers, who worked under the protection of Anubis, may have worn a wooden or terracotta mask fashioned in the image of the jackal-headed god. From the tomb of Sennutem at Deir el-Medina.

with a carefully specified procedure in seven successive stages, following the reception of the body by the priests, two or three days after death, on the east bank of the Nile. The corpse was then carried by boat across to the west bank, where it was installed in a "tent of purification" *(ibu)* presided over by the chief of embalmers, who bore the title "overseer *(imy-r)* of the mysteries."[12] As a representative of the god Anubis he may have worn a wooden or terracotta mask emblazoned with the god's image, and he was assisted in his duties by a lector priest responsible for the religious portion of the mummification ceremonies and the reading out of incantatory formulas.

The body was first stripped of clothing and thoroughly washed with natron in a water solution, then depilated, except for the hair of the head. Once dry, it was cleaned with a cloth that had been saturated with a coloring agent, probably an antiseptic dye, which left a fine reddish film on the skin. This explains the different epidermal shades that we find on mummies today.

The second step involved extraction of the brain through the nasal fossae, an operation performed on almost all the mummies of the New Kingdom.[13] The embalmer began by piercing the thin osseous wall of the cranial cavity with a sharp instrument plunged upward through the nostril. Using a long hook, he cut the brain into small pieces that he then pulled out through the nasal cavity. A preparation made from the ashes of plants such as prickly saltwort *(Salsola kali)* and mixed with soda (sodium carbonate) was next introduced in order to thoroughly clean the walls of the skull. After several hours the body was turned on its side or over onto its belly, with the head bent forward (the reason for the cervical fractures noted in a certain number of mummies) so that the residue would drain out. After a final washing the priest poured into the nostrils a hot resinous fluid and rotated the head several times so that the fluid completely covered the endocranial walls. The excess resin flowed downward into the occipital region, forming the classic "shield" described by radiologists. Finally, the orifices—nostrils, mouth, and ears—were covered with resin or melted wax, or plugged with wads of linen soaked in these substances.

In the third step, the abdominal and thoracic cavities were eviscerated through an incision whose location was modified over time. At first the opening was made parallel to the left flank below the lower edge of the ribs; later, during the reign of Thutmose III, it was placed farther down, parallel to the ileopubic line, though still on the left side.[14] A scribe (called *grammateus* in Diodorus 1.91) marked out the exact placement of the incision while the cutter *(paraschistes)* made the opening with a long curved knife of obsidian, the "Ethiopian stone" mentioned by

A bronze embalmer's knife from the New Kingdom with the figure of Anubis seated on a handle shaped like a papyrus plant that bears the name of the owner, Minmesout. According to Herodotus, incisions were usually made with a sharp curved knife of "Ethiopian stone," or obsidian. The Louvre, Paris.

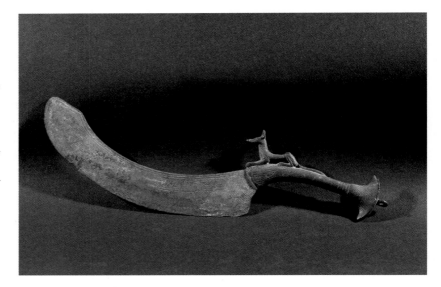

Herodotus (2.86). Through this rather narrow opening, about twelve centimeters wide on average, the embalmer (Herodotus, 2.85–89, calls him *taricheutes*—literally, "pickler"), standing on the cadaver's left side, inserted his left hand and, with this alone or with the aid of a small sharp stone, extracted the intestines, stomach, and liver, leaving the spleen and the kidneys in place as well as the bladder and the female genital organs.[15] (Male and female genitals alike were always left untouched so that the person's sexual life would be intact in the hereafter: if the phallus had been cut off it was wrapped in linen cloth and placed in the abdomen.) The diaphragm was then cut open in order to remove the lungs, but the heart, which was supposed to be the seat of consciousness and the sentiments, was left in the chest. If taken out by mistake, it was carefully put back and reattached.

The fourth step consisted in carefully washing the viscera with slightly nitrated water, then salting them and exposing them to the sun for a short time. They were then immersed in a sweet, strong liquid infused with aromatics and resin, known as *shedeh*, a highly alcoholic brew (about 40 proof) whose essential ingredient was fortified wine from the oases of the Libyan desert. The viscera were next imbued with fragrances—myrrh, turpentine resin, laudanum, and styrax (though almost surely not the "palm wine" mentioned by Herodotus and Diodorus)—before being coated with resin and oil. Each organ was then wrapped in a linen cloth and placed in one of four canopic vases.[16]

The embalmers now proceeded, in a fifth step, to dehydrate the body tissues. They began by filling the abdominal and thoracic cavities with cloth packets containing solid natron, linen wads impregnated with scented gum resin, and plant scraps such as straw and palm fibers, and then covering the whole body with great quantities of dry crystallized natron (ten times the volume of the body), which drew out water from the tissues by osmosis. The body was placed on a bed, tilted at a slight downward angle so that the residual fluids would drain into a container, with the result that 30 to 40 percent of its weight was lost. According to Herodotus (2.86) this step took seventy days, but the length of the process of dehydration remains a matter of controversy.[17]

The sixth step was inaugurated by the transfer of the body to another place—the "house of perfection" (per nefer)—where it was washed and cleaned, then coated with an oily liquid that gave it a reddish-orange tint. A mixture of fatty plant substances (juniper oil, cedar oil, bay leaf, pepper, rock rose, juniper berries) and milk, wine, and beeswax was then applied to restore a certain flexibility. Next the embalmers stuffed the body with various materials: linen soaked in resin, natron, lichen, onions, and mud, as well as a mixture of sawdust and pitch. The abdominal incision was typically sealed with wax (in kings it was concealed by a plate of metal or gold on which the wedjat-eye was engraved as a sign of protection and healing). The eyes were dried out with natron. Often they were removed, and sometimes replaced with cloth wadding (as, for example, in the case of Rameses III), precious stones, decorated prostheses, and even painted onions (Rameses IV). The nasal orifices were generally plugged up with cloth or wax.

In the seventh and final step, "keepers of mummies" (coachytes) worked for at least two weeks to bandage the mummy to the accompaniment of ritual acts and formulas. Between the layers of bandages, coated with wax and gum, they inserted protective amulets as well as jewels (143 in the case of Tutankhamun).[18] Once the body had been wrapped in a sturdy cloth shroud, a mask made of linen or papyrus and reinforced by plaster and resin was placed over the face and shoulders.

Fragrances, ointments, and resin were then poured over the finished mummy.

In addition to this elaborate form of mummification, which was reserved for members of the upper class, two less expensive and more expeditious types of embalming were common. For the poorest people the procedure was limited to injecting *syrmaia,* a juice extracted from radishes, into the intestines and then drying out the body in a natron bath. An intermediate form of mummification consisted in injecting oil of cedar into the abdomen before plunging the corpse into the natron solution. When the body was removed from the bath the oil was drained off, carrying with it the internal organs that it had liquefied. The deceased person was then returned to his family.[19]

4 The Modern Study of Mummies

Mummies have been an object of lively interest since ancient times. At first this interest was strictly a matter of personal enrichment or economic utility: mummies were sought not only for the valuable objects they contained but also for their use in pharmaceutical preparations and, in agriculture, as fertilizer. The robbing of graves by unscrupulous persons is a very old phenomenon. Thefts committed in the vicinity of Thebes were reported even during the reign of Rameses IX.[1]

It was not until the late nineteenth century that mummies were studied scientifically. In 1820 there took place in London a highly publicized dissection of a fifty-five-year-old woman from the 27th Dynasty,[2] but although this and similar procedures were informed by a knowledge of medicine, they were not scientific in the modern sense. Throughout most of that century the unbandaging of mummies was notable mainly for the morbid interest it aroused in a thrill-seeking public. The first detailed autopsies were conducted in 1886, following the discovery of the mummies of the most famous pharaohs at Deir el-Bahri. From that time onward dissections became more frequent and involved anthropologists, Egyptologists, and physicians. Yet even these studies, whose purpose was more demonstrative than scientific, were hardly rigorous. Hastily carried out, using crude and disfiguring methods, they produced relatively little information of lasting value.

It was only with Marc Armand Ruffer's work in the early 1920s that the discipline of paleopathology can really be said to have begun. And only since the 1970s have mummies been examined by multidisciplinary teams using noninvasive or otherwise minimally damaging

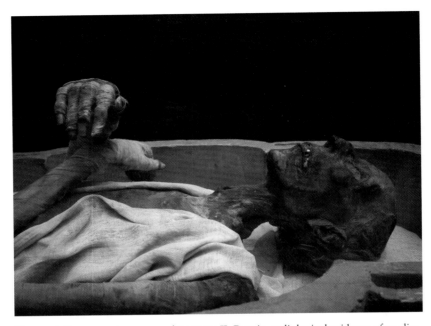

The partially wrapped mummy of Rameses II. Despite radiological evidence of cardio-vascular disease, this pharaoh lived to be at least eighty years old. Egyptian Museum, Cairo.

methods. The finest illustration is the analysis done in 1976 in Paris of the mummy of Rameses II by an extraordinary team of radiologists, dentists, anatomopathologists, parasitologists, bacteriologists, entomologists, and paleobotanists.[3]

Methods of
Analysis

One may well imagine the amazement of the patients and staff of the Cairo Hospital, home to the only X-ray machine in all of Egypt, at the sight of two resident English scholars, Elliot Smith and Wood Jones, handling the mummy of Thutmose III with extreme care as they got out of a taxi in front of the hospital in 1903. Egyptologists had very quickly understood the value of radiography, pioneered by Walter König, Thurston Holland, and Flinders Petrie, which had the advantage of leaving a mummy wrapped in bandages intact.[4] In 1913 Mario

Bertolotti reported the first osseous anomaly in a mummy of the 11th Dynasty. In 1931 another pioneer of the radiographic method, Roy Lee Moodie, published the results of a major examination of seventeen mummies. His study was largely superseded by that of P. H. Gray, who in 1967 described some two hundred observations of mummies preserved in various European museums, notably in Great Britain (London, Newcastle, and Liverpool) and the Netherlands. The following year the Egyptian government approved the radiographic examination of mummies conserved in the Cairo Museum by a team of experts from the University of Michigan.[5]

The appeal of conventional radiography, well summarized by both Don Brothwell and Maurice Bucaille, lay in its ability to detect the presence (or absence) of human remains beneath the bandages. It therefore held out the prospect, among others, of identifying the many bogus mummies produced by unscrupulous Egyptian dealers, especially in the nineteenth century, in response to rising demand from collectors. In addition to providing a wealth of anthropological information, X-rays made it possible to discover foreign bodies, particularly amulets, that had been hidden inside the bandages.[6]

It was now possible to estimate the height of a subject by examining the spinal column and the long bones of the limbs, and to determine its sex from images of the pelvis and the skull. X-rays of the jaw allowed a subject's age to be inferred from the mineralization of the teeth and the extent of dental eruption, while analysis of the skeleton as a whole, the skull, and the pelvis revealed the body's state of ossification, the synostosis of cranial sutures and obliteration of the fontanels (that is, the extent to which the "soft spots" in the skull had closed), and the surface area of the symphysis pubis and the sacroiliac articulation. Thus dental radiology has yielded an approximate age of death for three pharaonic mummies: Thutmose II (30–40 years), Merenptah (60–70 years), and Rameses II (85–90 years). Radiological examination of the bones of Thutmose I put his age at only 18 years, in contradiction of the traditional account, according to which he died at about 50 years of age after a reign lasting 11 years and 9 months—unless, of course, the mummified body has been misidentified.[7]

Radiography also made it possible to detect osseous pathology—abnormalities or diseases of the bones—which could then be analyzed further, if necessary, by more specialized techniques. X-rays of the lower spine of Amenhotep II, for example, showed a narrowing of the sacroiliac interspaces and calcification of the dorsolumbar paraspinal ligaments, suggesting a diagnosis of the rheumatic disease ankylosing spondylitis. Lesions of the soft tissues were also discovered (arterial calcifications, biliary lithiases, calcified cysts, and so on) for which no explanation has yet been found.[8]

Xeroradiography, a related but less well known technique that was highly regarded before the advent of the computerized axial tomography (CAT) scanner, has also been applied to the study of mummies. Because it records the image produced by X-rays with the aid of photoelectric methods, it has the advantage of giving high-definition pictures of the details of the soft tissues and cartilage.[9]

Polytome tomography, likewise used mostly before the advent of the CAT scanner, made it possible to obtain cross-sectional images of mummies, layer by layer, by scanning X-rays. Using this very fruitful technique to study the complex bony structures of the cranium, a team led by Aidan Cockburn was able in 1969 to examine the orifice (invisible in standard images) through which the contents of the cranial cavity were removed.[10]

But it was the introduction of the CAT scanner in 1972 that really revolutionized the study of mummies. In 1977 this technique was applied for the first time by Derek Harwood-Nash and his team from Toronto in order to analyze a mummy dating from the 22nd Dynasty (about 900 B.C.). Between 1978 and 1981, members of the department of anthropology and human genetics at the University of Tübingen, working under the direction of Wolfgang Pahl, along with researchers in the department of medical radiology there, undertook scanographic investigations of mummies not only from Egypt but also from South America and Asia. Most important of all were the many tomodensitometric analyses made during the 1980s by Theo Falke and Myron Marx, which yielded a great deal of valuable paleopathological information.[11]

The advantage of CAT scanning over other techniques is that, by providing very fine cross-sections of the whole body, it allows the skeleton, muscular masses, and contents of the thoracic and abdominal cavities to be inspected in precise detail. To name but one example,

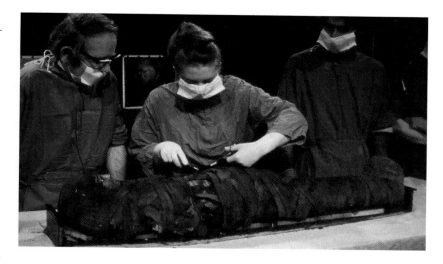

Rosalie David and her team begin an autopsy of Manchester mummy 1770 in 1975. Radiography revealed the calcified remains of a male Guinea worm in the mummy's abdominal wall. The lower legs had been amputated, probably about two weeks before death, perhaps as a result of an unsuccessful attempt to extract female Guinea worms, which sometimes try to break out through the skin of the legs.

a scanographic study of Lady Tashat (daughter of Djehutyhotep and "guardian of the gates of the temple of Amun" at Thebes during the 25th Dynasty) succeeded in reconstructing a magnificent image of her heart in which structures corresponding to the cords and papillary muscles are clearly visible in the residual ventricular chamber.[12] This kind of investigation also throws valuable light on the mode of bandaging employed, funerary objects hidden beneath the bandages, substances placed within the body, the shape, size, and exact location of the incision in the abdominal wall, and especially the techniques of mummification applied (complete or partial evisceration, the material used for subcutaneous padding, the kind of artificial eyes inserted, and so on).

Tomodensitometric analysis has recently been extended by three-dimensional reconstruction, notably in the case of a priestess of the 22nd Dynasty named Tjentmutengebtiu, who is preserved in her sarcophagus at the British Museum in London. X-ray computer tomography of the mummified tissues enabled researchers to reconstruct her head and even the expression of the face, without removing the body from its sarcophagus or even touching the bandages. Images of the teeth placed her age at death between 19 and 23 years, whereas the archaeological data had suggested an age between 25 and 40 years. Applied to three other mummies at the Manchester Museum in England, this tech-

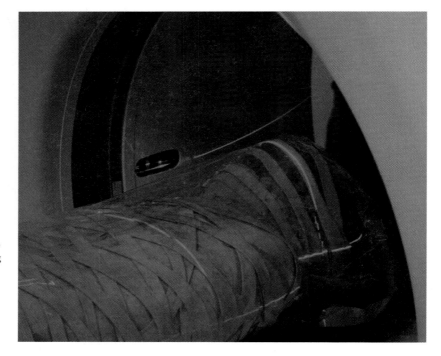

An anonymous mummy being placed in a CAT scanner in the CT-3D Advanced Imaging Lab at Beth Israel Deaconess Medical Center in Boston. The three-dimensional images produced by computerized axial tomography make it possible to determine the body's probable age, gender, and state of health at the time of death—without exposing the mummy to invasive or disfiguring procedures.

nique has yielded images bearing a striking resemblance to statuettes depicting the same people.[13]

Nuclear magnetic resonance imaging, by contrast, has been of little assistance in this connection, mainly because the dehydration involved in the process of mummification prevents protons from being generated.[14]

Preliminary Examination

The use of standard radiology and scanning to determine the morphological and anatomical characteristics of the subject, normal and pathological alike, is indispensable to a successful autopsy.

Before the actual dissection begins, the body is inspected for lesions of the skin, which resembles a dark, cracked shell because of the resins and waxes applied by the embalmers. Preliminary examination of the mummy of Thutmose II, for example, revealed the presence of cutaneous bumps (papules) between one millimeter and one centimeter high on the chest, shoulders, arms, hands, buttocks, legs, and feet; only the skin of the face, palms, and soles of the feet was unmarked.[15] Two hypothetical diagnoses of these dermatological disorders have been proposed, namely that the pharaoh presents evidence of either metabolic dysfunction—even xanthomas, cutaneous amyloidosis, and papular mucinosis—or Darier's disease (keratosis follicularis). The diffuse aspect of the lesions and of the calcifications of the soft tissues, as well as the pharaoh's young age and frail constitution, tend to favor the first hypothesis. The topography of the papules, however, and the presence of the same features in the son and grandson of Thutmose II, suggest a family disease and point instead toward the second diagnosis. Additionally, examination of the mummy of Rameses V, a pharaoh who died at about the age of 30, disclosed papules on the face, abdomen, and thighs that are commonly accepted as smallpox scars, though it has not been possible to establish a definitive diagnosis in the absence of a complete anatomicopathological examination.[16]

Four mummies that exhibit tattooed points and strokes arranged in parallel or diamond-shaped lines have been analyzed: Amunet (a priestess of Hathor found in a tomb from the 11th Dynasty), two Theban dancers from a later period, and a Nubian woman. The priestess of Hathor, for example, was tattooed on her left shoulder, right arm, right thigh, and inguinal region, as well as on the abdomen above the navel; a large ellipse was inscribed in the region above the pubis. Examination of the face in many mummies discloses a deformation and a lengthening related to the process of mummification, during which the jaw was restored to its normal position with more or less difficulty. It sometimes happens that the nose, frequently broken during embalming, is missing and the nasal cavity has been equipped with a prosthesis. The earlobes of certain mummies have been pierced and deformed by the weight of earrings: in the case of one male adolescent, ears made of resin and cotton tissue have been found, though it was not possible to determine whether they were attached before or after death.[17]

| Endoscopic Analysis | In a second phase the inside of the mummy is studied by means of a classic anatomical dissection that is similar in every respect to the ones performed today by medical students. Increasingly, however, endoscopy is employed before dissection. Derek Notman and Michelle Stanworth |

of the Manchester Museum Mummy Project have demonstrated the value of this technique, which is continually being improved by the miniaturization of fibroscopic probes. It enables researchers not only to examine lesions of the abdomen and thorax but also to explore these cavities, assess the technique of embalming employed, and inspect organs and the contents of canopic jars. Its chief advantage is that it permits detailed structural and chemical analysis of tissues.[18] For this purpose the probe is introduced through the embalmer's abdominal incision rather than through the natural oral and anal orifices, which typically have been plugged up. The head can also be explored endoscopically through the external auditory canals, and in certain cases a biopsy of brain tissue can be carried out as well.

Tissue Studies

The major obstacle to tissue studies used to be the dehydration of mummified tissues, which made the slicing of very fine sections of tissue and their microscopic examination difficult. Following an unsuccessful attempt to rehydrate tissues by Johann Czermak in 1852, S. G. Shattock obtained certain preliminary results a half century later by freezing fragments of the aorta of Merenptah. But it was Ruffer, more than anyone else, who was responsible for advancing histological knowledge. In 1910 he developed a new method of rehydration, soaking tissue samples for 34–48 hours in a mixture of 1 percent sodium carbonate solution and formalin. Over the following decades research continued. Finally, in 1955, A. T. Sandison succeeded in perfecting a technique for the preparation of mummified tissues that opened up the way for interesting work to be done.[19] The majority of these tissues could now be subjected to proper examination: though some tissues, such as those of muscles, the liver, and nerves, generally exhibit considerable alteration, others have survived the process of mummification in perfect condition and yield very fine images, such as the skin and superficial body growth (hair, nails, teeth, and so on), cartilaginous tissues, vessels, and blood cells.[20]

In 1968 the first scanning studies performed by electron microscopy on bits of skin from two Predynastic mummies (ca. 4000 B.C.) showed that the epidermis had been preserved but without any visible cell nuclei. From this it was concluded that the mummies' state of preservation was due to the very dry climate rather than to the embalming process, which was thought to expose the epidermis to abrasion on account of the natron solutions it involved. In 1993, however, an ultrastructural study of the skin of two Egyptian mummies (ca. 150 B.C. and 90 B.C.)[21] discovered, in addition to spores and bacteria, perfectly preserved cutaneous structures, in particular the epidermal desmosomes, intercellular junctions, and the fibrillar components of the extracellular matrix of the dermis. These results confirmed the excellence of the embalming procedures employed.

Dietary Analysis

We know something about the diet of the Egyptians from the images on the walls of their tombs. The best-known feast is the one discovered by the English archaeologist Bryan Emery, in tomb 30 at Saqqara, dating from the 2nd Dynasty (about 2700 B.C.), which included a fish, a roasted quail, pigeon stew, and kidneys accompanied by bread and honey cakes as well as jujube berries and stewed figs, all washed down with wine. Archaeologists today are increasingly interested in the analysis of feces and coprolites recovered from mummies after dissection of the intestines.[22] Microscopic examination of these substances, after rehydration, discloses their constituent elements and could in principle, as part of an analysis of a homogeneous series of specimens, furnish precise data about the dietary habits of the population as a whole. It is not always possible to recover such material, however, since its preservation within the body by embalming depends on the type of procedure employed and the period. The subjects analyzed to date do not constitute a sufficiently large and uniform group to allow extrapolation of broad patterns of consumption. Individual results are nonetheless suggestive. The presence of vegetable fibers in the feces of Henhenet (wife of Mentuhotep II), for example, and of muscular fibers in those of PUM II (an Egyptian mummy of the Ptolemaic Period dating from about 170 B.C. and preserved at the University of Pennsylvania Museum) has made it possible to determine the contents of their last meals.[23]

Ancillary evidence has been provided by the analysis of depilated hairs from the scalp, the face, and the rest of the body, along with their follicles, by means of optic and electron microscopy. Thus, for example, it has been possible to establish that Rameses II was a redhead. More generally, it has been possible to assign mummified subjects to particular population groups on the basis of data about hair growth, as well as the form and color of individual hairs. Lesions compatible with pathologies of the scalp have also been noted, principally ringworm due to dermatophytic fungi. Spectrometric examination of head and body hair has enabled researchers to identify a certain number of mineral and toxic substances, among these significant concentrations of trace elements. Sizable amounts of calcium, magnesium, strontium, manganese, zinc, iron, and copper have been found in 168 mummies. Related studies have explained differential concentrations of minerals by reference to dietary habits, and findings of the presence of certain drugs in the hair of mummies have consistently been verified by different teams of researchers.[24]

Dating Techniques

Two methods, radiocarbon dating and amino acid racemization, are employed to establish the age of mummies. The first method, developed by Willard F. Libby in 1947, consists in measuring the radioactivity of carbon-14 in mummy muscle samples.[25] It depends on the fact that the activity of this isotope, which has a half-life of about 5,730 years and is permanently incorporated by any organism that absorbs carbon dioxide contaminated by cosmic rays, regularly diminishes as a function of time. Measuring the level of radioactivity of carbon-14 with a Geiger counter therefore makes it possible to calculate the time elapsed since the death of an organism. The advantage of this method is that it can be used for any structure containing carbon that is between 100 and 40,000 years old. The disadvantage is that sources of error are many since the results depend on the volume of the sample and are vulnerable to contamination by neighboring elements. Accordingly, carbon-14 dating is useful mainly for obtaining an approximate idea of an object's age.

The second method exploits a technique developed by Robin A. Barraco in 1973, based on a reaction known as racemization that occurs in amino acids.[26] These synthesizing elements make up the proteins of living beings and rotate the plane of polarization of plane-polarized light passing through them. Because some rotate the plane of polarized light toward the left, some toward the right, and because the ratio of the two changes over time, it is possible to deduce the age of a given tissue by studying that ratio. The advantage of this method is that it requires only a small amount of material. The disadvantage is that its results vary as a function of temperature. In the case of mummies, its usefulness depends on knowing, at least approximately, the thermal conditions under which they were buried.

Paleoserology

The study of blood groups was extended to paleoserology for the first time in 1927 by Kritchevsky, who demonstrated the presence of substances called Landsteiner agglutinogens A and B in cadavers. L. G. Boyd, studying the blood groups of Egyptian mummies, noted the frequency of groups A, B, and O in ancient Egypt, which turns out to be substantially the same as what one finds in that country today. Moreover, the presence of group B in Predynastic mummies going back beyond 3000 B.C. argued against the suggestion that group B was only a mutation of group O that had appeared during the Christian era. Subsequent analysis confirmed among other things the kinship of the unknown royal male from tomb KV55 in the Valley of the Kings (perhaps Smenkhkara) and Tutankhamun.[27]

The human leukocyte antigen (HLA) group, which is known to play an essential role in tissue compatibility and the genetic predisposition to certain afflictions, has also been detected in samples of muscle and of hypodermic tissue (the connective tissue under the skin). This result opens up a particularly promising avenue for research in organic paleopathology, which may make it possible one day to identify genetic diseases that until now have been unknown or only suspected among the ancient Egyptians. In principle the study of the HLA group will also enable anthropologists to obtain more precise information about the origin of populations and their development. For the moment, however, considerations of cost and technical difficulty have worked to limit its use.

Microbiology and Biochemistry

Microbiological research has isolated a number of microorganisms in the bodies of mummies. In the lungs of two mummies Ruffer discovered a bacterial agent similar to the pneumonia-causing pneumococcus and a gram-negative bacterium similar to the plague bacillus *(Yersinia pestis)*. In 1977 a team of researchers at the Royal Ontario Museum in Canada isolated calcified eggs of worms responsible for schistosomiasis (bilharziasis) in the liver, intestines, and kidneys of a weaver named Nakht (conventionally referred to as ROM 1) who had been dead for thirty-two centuries. This same mummy was also a host for tapeworm eggs in the intestines and *Trichinella spiralis* cysts in the intercostal muscles. A team from the University of Pennsylvania Museum led by Aidan Cockburn found an *Ascaris lumbricoides* egg in the intestine of a priest from the Ptolemaic period, the aforementioned PUM II.[28] Moreover, the *Para*Sight™-F test, which is based on the ELISA method, has been applied to fragments of skin, muscle, and lung tissue from four Predynastic mummies as well as several embalmed mummies (two dating from the 20th Dynasty, one from the 25th Dynasty, and another from the Nubian Ballana Period, A.D. 350–550), all of which show the presence of an antigen characteristic of *Plasmodium falciparum*, the agent responsible for malaria.[29]

In the realm of the infinitely small one proceeds next to paleobiochemistry, which analyzes both organic macromolecular components (proteins, lipids, carbohydrates) and proportions of simple chemical elements. The identification of proteins in terms of their molecular weight and constituent amino acids yields valuable information not only about the preservation of mummified tissues but also, since natron has the property of stabilizing proteins of high molecular weight, about the results of embalming. Insight into different types of diet may be obtained from the study of lipids, carbohydrates, and vitamins, while research into cholesterol levels, triglycerides, phospholipids, and vitamin E casts further light upon styles of living in ancient Egypt. The proportion of chemical elements (sodium, potassium, calcium, and magnesium, as well as lead, mercury, silver, and so on) in mummified remains can be discovered by means of atomic absorption spectrophotometry. Thus, for example, comparative studies of mummies and present-day human beings have shown identical concentrations of mercury in the bones, by contrast with lead, whose concentrations are thirty times less in mummies.[30]

During the second half of the 1980s Svante Pääbo pioneered the application of techniques in molecular biology to the domain of paleopathology, opening up extremely interesting possibilities. In 1985 Pääbo identified strands of ancient DNA in histological preparations taken from striated skeletal muscle and connective tissue in mummified corpses of the pharaonic era. He went on to isolate genetic material in samples taken from 23 Egyptian mummies of different periods, and to extract and clone a fragment of DNA of 3.4 kilobases from the mummy of a child dating from about 500 B.C. and preserved in the Aegyptisches Museum in Berlin. The proportion of a specific cardiac enzyme discovered in the mummy of Horem Kenisi, priest of Amun, who died at about the age of 60 around 1050 B.C., suggested a retrospective diagnosis of myocardial infarction.[31]

Paleobiochemistry, in its several branches, holds out the prospect of being able to understand the frequency and evolution of previously unknown diseases in ancient Egypt. In addition to illuminating kinship relations among family members of the pharaohs, it may help us trace patterns of migration among the inhabitants of the Nile Valley and neighboring peoples during the pharaonic era.[32]

PART III

FROM CRADLE TO GRAVE

5 Mothers and Children

The place of women in Egyptian society has been succinctly described by Christiane Desroches-Noblecourt: "The feminine image represents love, woman as mother, weeper (or mourner), one who stimulates desire, who gives life and watches over the deceased on their departure for eternity. In these essential roles she appears desirable, respectable, and protective: in all of them she embodies attraction, need, comfort."[1]

Wife and Mother

Pictorial and other representations of Egyptian women in the company of their husbands during various festivities testify to the crucial place they held in daily life. Yet one cannot quite speak of an equality of the sexes, as Pierre Grandet observes: "Neither angels nor demons, but simply men, the ancient Egyptians, as individuals, felt toward women the feelings they have always inspired in men: love and hate, desire and jealousy, respect and scorn. Lively though these passions were, as a society they considered maternity to be a woman's exclusive vocation, and monogamous marriage the primary occasion for her development." Female health was therefore considered mainly a matter of the well-being of a future wife and mother—two functions that *The Instructions of Any,* a Ramessid wisdom text concerning the purpose of the family that dates from the 19th or 20th Dynasty, insists were closely linked: "Take a wife while you are young, that she may give you a son. May she give birth for you while you are young. It is wise to have progeny. A man is in a good [position] whose people are numerous: he is honored in proportion to his children."[2]

In a society that was essentially monogamous, despite a few cases of official bigamy, each couple was expected to have several children, preferably boys, in order to preserve social respectability and to avoid disgrace: the opposite was seen as proof of egotism.[3] In addition to children there were parents to be cared for (a widowed mother, for example, or a sick father), a sister still too young to marry, and so on. Taken together they made up the large families depicted on Egyptian funerary monuments.

Fertility and Pregnancy Testing

In this social context, inability to have children carried the risk of repudiation[4] and, moreover, was experienced as a sign of divine disfavor, one that young women feared more than anything else—and for which they alone were held responsible. In the event of a problematic delivery, for example, blame fell wholly upon them, not upon the gods. To ward off infertility adolescent girls wore belts decorated with gold threads in a cowrie pattern symbolizing the vulva. Such accessories were found mainly among daughters of wealthy families. But other amulets representing a child, a pregnant woman, or the god Bes were popular as well, all of them thought to be capable of conferring fertility on those who wore them.

If infertility was confirmed, recourse could be had to magic. An original procedure for diagnosing this condition is described in Carlsberg IV: "To determine who will bear and who will not bear: you should place an onion bulb deep in her flesh [that is, vagina], leaving it there all night until dawn. If the odour of it appears in her mouth she will give birth, if it does not she will never give birth."[5] This test assumed an unobstructed path between the vagina and the upper digestive tract: the rising up of the odor of the onion from the genital organs to the mouth confirmed that the body's canals, or vessels *(metu)*, were clear. Infertility was supposed by the Egyptians to cut off communication between the genitals and the rest of the organism: difficult deliveries, among other things, might result from the obstruction of these vessels. This notion was later to become influential. Indeed, the procedure described in the papyrus was adopted by the Greeks, who incorporated it into the diagnosis of sterility contained in the Hippocratic treatise *Sterile Women*. Subsequently it was adopted by the Arabs as well.[6]

So long as she was fertile a woman could fulfill her role as mother, beginning with the conception of a child. She shared this task with the father, of course, but also with the potter god Khnum, who actively collaborated in procreation and exerted a fundamental influence over it. In the course of embryonic life the dynamic breath of the god mingled with the blood of the mother, the carrier of life, in order to bind the seed, believed to be extracted from the bone of the father, thus creating the skeleton of the infant.[7] The mother, in this philosophical and religious account, contributed the non-osseous part of the child. In her uterus (*mut remetj*—literally, "mother of mankind"), which the Egyptians described as a wandering, unattached organ, flesh deposited itself on the incipient skeleton laid down by the father.[8] This flesh was thought to be partly composed of mother's milk, itself produced by the liquefaction of her tissues during pregnancy.

For the Egyptians it was the quality of this milk that determined the sex of the child: the best milk yielded a boy (in several remedies it is described as "milk of a woman who has brought a boy into the world"). The pressure to produce male offspring led the Egyptians to do everything possible to discover the sex of the child before birth. To determine this one might, for example, take "barley [and] emmer [hard wheat] that the woman has moistened with her urine, each day, as well as with dates and sand, [placed] in two [separate] sacks. If together they grow she will give birth [in the normal way]. If [only] the barley grows, this signifies a male child. If [only] the wheat grows, this signifies a girl. If they do not grow, she will not give birth [in the normal way]" (Berlin 199).

What was the reasoning behind this strange test? It is difficult to say. Two linguistic interpretations have been proposed. The first rests on the phonetic identity of the words "father" and "barley" (both being pronounced *it* in Egyptian), and therefore on the coincidence between the grain and the male genital organ; the second, due to Grapow, on the fact that "barley" in Egyptian grammar is masculine in gender, whereas "wheat" is feminine. A third hypothesis, advanced by Jürgen Thorwald, assigns a pragmatic origin to this recipe on the basis of an observation made by Julius Manger, a researcher in the laboratory of the Institute of Pharmacology at Würzburg, who in 1933 noticed a more rapid rate of growth in wheat mixed with the urine of a woman pregnant with a boy, and in barley, again mixed with urine, when the fetus was a girl—in contradiction of the text in the Berlin papyrus. Another interesting study, published thirty years later, showed that seeds of wheat and barley moistened with the urine of a pregnant woman germinated in 40 percent of the cases studied.[9] One wonders whether the ancient Egyptian prescription was merely a coincidence or whether it was due to a keen talent for observation.

Calculating
the Length
of Pregnancy

Two texts from the Roman Period, found in a temple at Esna, mention a curious detail concerning the term of pregnancy, referring to the needs of the fetus over "ten months." How is such a long gestation to be explained? Are we to assume that its onset was diagnosed in a random manner? To be sure, we do not know whether the Egyptians considered amenorrhea, the absence of the menses, as an obvious sign of pregnancy. But their diagnosis depended on careful examination of the skin, breasts, and venous system, described in the Berlin and Kahun papyri—observations that Hippocrates himself was to endorse in his aphorisms. The surprising length of pregnancy can be accounted for on other grounds, and very simply, by reference to the calendar: the Egyptians calculated the passing of time in lunar months of twenty-eight days each, and counted a partial month as a full month.[10]

With the end of ten such periods, then, a pregnancy would have reached its term. For protection, pregnant women wore amulets made of ivory and other materials throughout their pregnancy, around the neck or the waist, representing divinities such as Bes, Taweret, and Anubis. Holes were also drilled in figurines of the goddess Taweret and articles of clothing attached to them. To ascertain whether delivery would occur without harmful consequences for the health of either the mother or the child, the Egyptians believed it was necessary to confirm the pregnant woman's vitality by examining her vessels, which guided the passage of divine breath through the body. Only this breath was capable of keeping the fetus alive—as the Berlin papyrus suggests, describing a test that could very well correspond to today's practice of taking the pulse:

> [Other means of] seeing. At her bed you will smear her breasts and
> both arms up to the shoulders with new oil. You shall rise early in the
> morning to see this. [If] you note that her vessels are whole and per-

Elaborate symbolic ritual, including incantations and the display of protective objects, surrounded the delivery of a child. This wooden amulet, showing a mother and her newborn, was used to ensure a safe and easy birth. British Museum.

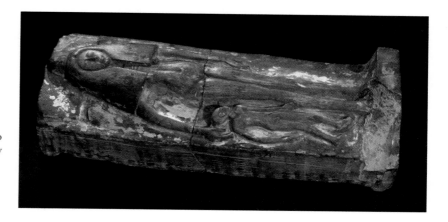

fect, none of them being sunken [that is, collapsed]: calm delivery. [If] you note that they are sunken and have the color [?] of her own skin, this signifies miscarriage [?]. [If] you note that they are whole [between] the night and [the moment of] their examination: she will deliver late.[11]

Another method for establishing a diagnosis, found in the Kahun papyrus, relies on examination of the skin after pressure is applied: "You must pinch the belly, the edge [?] of your thumb being placed above her fetus [*menia*, literally "that which beats"]. [If] . . . [it] comes apart [that is, if the mark disappears], [she will give birth in the normal way]. [If] it does not disappear, she will not give birth [in the normal way], nor ever again" (Kahun 29).

Various signs allowing the physician to predict a normal delivery are found in these same papyri, from the firmness of the breasts to the vomiting of a pregnant woman smeared with the dregs or lees of beer (the number of vomitings corresponding to the number of children she will deliver).

Giving Birth

Delivery of the child involved a mixture of religious and magical practices, on the one hand, and medical techniques, on the other. Early in the pharaonic period, during the 6th Dynasty, a primitive seat or birthing stool *(meskhenet)* consisting of three bricks was used to help release the infant from the mother's body. From the 18th Dynasty onward, a true obstetrical stool, or, in the case of certain privileged persons, a low seat, replaced this rudimentary device. Since the vertex, or head-down, presentation of the baby was considered normal (the hieroglyph representing childbirth shows the head and the two arms of the fetus reaching out of the mother's belly), delivery always occurred in the squatting position.[12]

But the symbolic interpretation of birth also greatly influenced the circumstances under which labor took place. Men were excluded from the birthing room. The mother-to-be was accompanied by several women who came to welcome the new being fashioned by Khnum, symbolically substituting themselves for the tutelary goddesses of birth. The first played the role of Nephthys and positioned herself behind the mother in order to hold her in place during labor. The second, standing in for Heqet, exhorted her to push, while the third, who represented Isis, was responsible for controlling the expulsion of the child from the womb and for receiving the infant. Surrounded by these helpers the mother recited prayers addressed to Khnum, invoking Shu, who symbolized the vital element breathed in by the newborn, and Amun, or Man: "Fear Khnum, pregnant women, [you] who have passed your term, for it is he, Shu, the god of birth, who opens up the lips of the feminine organ and, in the guise of Amun, brings about birth."[13]

The process of giving birth did not end with delivery. It remained to expel the placenta, which was considered the twin brother of the newborn child and so possessed great symbolic value. For this reason it was either buried in the garden of the house or, having been carefully preserved, was used to cure the child in times of sickness and to cauterize deep wounds. Afterward the mother was subjected to a period of fourteen days of "purification" away from her house—a rite similar to that of the Hebrews, as it is described in Leviticus 12:2–5: "If a woman conceives, and bears a male child, then she shall be unclean seven days . . . But if she bears a female child, then she shall be unclean two weeks."

We know from certain mummies, however, that not all births were as uneventful as this account may suggest. Thus the corpse of Henhenet (wife of Mentuhotep II), who had a very narrow pelvis, exhibits traces of a tear of the vulva over its entire length together with a broad vesico-vaginal fistula—an abnormal connection between the bladder and the vagina. Even more striking is the mummy of a woman who died in childbirth, found lying on her back, thighs spread apart and knees bent: her newborn is dead, its head crushed.[14]

To facilitate birth and to ease difficult deliveries, the Egyptians used various methods in addition to placing an article of clothing on a statuette of Taweret. A preparation might, for example, be administered during or after labor: "Another remedy for delivering: sea salt: 1; emmer, 1; female [?] rush: 1. Dress the lower part of the belly with it" (Ebers 800). Other remedies were employed to help expel the placenta: "Remedy to cause the placenta of a woman to go down to its natural place: pine sawdust. Put this in dregs. Smear [this mixture over] brick covered with tissue and have her sit upon it" (Ebers 789).[15]

Newborns

Once washed, dried, and placed in a sort of cradle made of brick, the newborn baby remained vulnerable. The first moments of life were carefully monitored and the infant's robustness assessed. A magical ritual was performed to protect the child before its name was chosen and its future predicted. Beyond this, the chief aspect of the medical and symbolic care of the newborn, aimed at guaranteeing its healthy development in the first three years of life, involved feeding.

Neonatal Care

No matter that it had been safely brought into the world, the newborn was hardly out of danger: rates of infant mortality were very high, and may have varied between 20 and 50 percent during the first year after birth. Infants were therefore carefully watched during the first hours and days after birth, with a view not only to gauging their resistance to illness but also to protecting them from it. Vigilance did not always meet with success—witness the many newborns and infants buried next to ancient houses in Illahun, some in coffins woven from fibers (or made of plastered layers of papyrus known as cartonnage) that were decorated for the occasion and adorned with protective amulets.[16]

Forecasts of survival formulated on the day of birth had a different basis. Some relied on signs still familiar to us today, such as the moaning of a baby suffering from hypotonia (low muscle tone), its face turned downward: "Another determination. If one hears a moaning voice, it means he will die. If he turns his face toward the ground, it too means he will die" (Ebers 839). Others rest on principles peculiar to ancient Egyptian medicine, such as the integrity of the body's vessels, which had already been crucial during the mother's pregnancy and during childbirth. Thus the newborn's reaction to being fed a bit of the placenta, the classic symbol of nourishment, provided evidence of its likely fate: "Another thing to be done for him on the day when he is brought into the world: a lump of his placenta, with [. . .]. You shall grind [this] up in some milk and it shall be given to him in a *henu*-vase. If he brings it up, this means he will die. If he [swallows] it, this means he will live" (Ramesseum IV, C, 17–24).

Still other principles remain obscure to us. No rational explanation has yet been found for the following test: "Another: to determine the fate of a child on the day he is brought into the world. If he says *ny*, it means he will live; if he says *embi*, it means he will die" (Ebers 838)—even though we know that *ny* and *embi* are translated respectively as "yes" and "no."

The vital diagnosis having been made, the newborn enjoyed the closest attention from members of the immediate family, who sought to protect it against harmful forces, earthly and divine alike. For example, one might "make an [amulet] for the personal protection of a child on the day when it is brought into the world: . . . a lump of feces on top, when [the child] has come down from the belly of his mother" (Ramesseum IV, C, 15–16). But incantations could also perform this function. The one that follows, evidently recited by the mother and her attendants, had the declared purpose of chasing away evil spirits. But nothing prevents us from supposing, along with Christiane Desroches-Noblecourt, that such prayers were also thought to act upon the young mother and, by lessening her anxiety, to promote lactation:[17]

> Your protection is the protection of the sky . . . of the earth . . . of the
> night . . . of the day . . .
> Your protection is the protection of the seven divine Entities,
> Who ordered the earth when it was uninhabited;
> And placed the heart in its right place . . .
> May each god protect your name,
> Every place where you will be,
> All milk that you will drink,

Every breast from which you will be fed,
Every knee on which you will be seated,
Every piece of clothing that will be put on you,
Every place where you will pass the day,
Every protection that will be uttered over you,
Every object on which you will be laid down,
Every knot that will be tied on you,
Every amulet that will be placed around your neck,
[May all of these things] protect you.
May you be kept in good health, by them
May you be kept safe, by them,
May you be soothed, by them, each god and each goddess.
Vanish, [demon, you] who come in darkness, who enter cunningly,
Your nose behind you, and your face turned backward,
[You] whom the reason of your coming shall escape!
Vanish, [specter, you] who come in darkness, who enter cunningly,
Your nose behind you, and your face turned backward,
[You] whom the reason of your coming shall escape!
Have you come to take this child in your arms?
I will not allow you to take him in your arms.
Have you come to calm him?
I will not allow you to calm him.
Have you come to do him harm?
I will not allow you to do him harm.
Have you come to take him away?
I will not allow you to take him away. (Berlin 3027)

Premature infants, particularly susceptible to early death, were not neglected. Another magical formula ("Incantation for an unfortunate woman who has delivered before term") was expressly intended for them:

Greetings to you [the seven threads of linen], by means of which Isis wove and Nephthys spun a [large] knot of divine fabric composed of seven knots. You shall be protected by it, O child!

[Henceforth] in good health, such a thread of such [a goddess] . . . shall make you healthy; it shall make you sound; it shall make every god, every goddess propitious for you; it shall strike down enemies, hostile creatures; it shall close the mouth of anyone who wishes you evil [?], as when the mouth was closed, as when the mouths of the 117 asses that were in the lake of Dedes were sealed; I know them, and so I know their names, but [the names] are not known of the one who would wish to harm this child to the point of making it ill . . .

One says this incantation four times over forty round pearls, seven smaragdine stones, seven pieces of gold, seven threads of linen woven [and spun] by two sisters of the womb [such as Isis and Nephthys]: the one wove, the other spun. May such an amulet be made from it with seven knots and may it be placed around the neck of the child: this shall protect its body. (Berlin 3027)

The final, decisive step in caring for the newborn, intended to ensure continuing soundness of body and mind once the signs of good health had been observed, was the giving of a name. In bestowing this "great" or "true name" upon a child, parents modified a divine or royal name and added to it a verb or an adjective.[18] In some cases the child received the name of a god or goddess called out by the mother herself at the moment of giving birth or upon coming out of a dream. According to legend, the name of a royal child was always uttered during the act of love in which the child was conceived, and whispered to the young queen by the goddesses who attended the delivery of her child.

Breastfeeding   "Give back to your mother twice the bread that she gave you, and carry her as she carried you. She often took care of you and did not put you down when you were born after ten months. She patiently suffered [to hold] her breast in your mouth for three years."[19] This passage from *The Instructions of Any* tells us a great deal about the care Egyptian mothers gave a newborn baby, to the point of breastfeeding the child for the first three years of its life. The mother generally kept the infant next to her throughout the day in a pouch fastened around her neck. Numerous statues and bas-reliefs attest to this, depicting a woman seated on the ground, one knee raised, feeding a newborn or, more often, a very young seated infant. Goddesses themselves figure in these scenes, typically Isis giving her breast to her child or to the pharaoh. These divine exemplars served to emphasize the crucial importance of breastfeeding, which no doubt explains the respect shown by wealthy families to the nurses in charge of feeding their children. One such nurse, who suckled Queen Hatshepsut, is venerated in the sanctuary of Hathor at Deir el-Bahri. This most natural of all forms of nourishment is an effective defense against rickets—which in ancient Egypt, at least as far as we are able to tell, was practically nonexistent.[20]

For these three long years, critical for the baby's survival and development, it was necessary to guarantee both the flow and the quality of maternal milk. To stimulate lactation Egyptian medicine relied on magical practices, notably the wearing of amulets bearing the likeness of Taweret, the hippopotamus goddess, accompanied by incantations and various formulas. Use was also made of hollow figurines, probably filled with milk that poured out through a hole in one of the nipples—a symbolic aid to breastfeeding. The recipes associated with this sort of treatment may seem to be of doubtful psychological effectiveness: "To bring milk back to a nurse whom a child suckles: the dorsal spine of a fighting fish. Boil [this] in fat/oil [*merhet*]. Smear her back with [it]" (Ebers 836). Another remedy consisted of "tainted barley bread, whose fire [for cooking] will have been prepared with *khesau*-plants. [It] is to be eaten by the woman whose legs are bent" (Ebers 837).[21]

The mother's milk, which the Egyptians saw as a potential carrier of disease, had to be monitored for quality. On this point physicians were punctilious: "Examination of bad milk: you shall examine its odor, similar to the stench of fish"—by contrast with that of potable milk, whose "odor is similar to that of the [tiger] nut" (Ebers 796).[22]

The baby's health was considered, then, to depend on that of its mother, who needed to be protected in her turn against various afflictions, especially chapping, inflammation, and swelling of the breasts. The Egyptians feared that, even where such pathologies did not actually stunt the child's growth by inhibiting lactation, they might alter the quality of the milk and transmit noxious substances to the child. To guard against the threat of infection an "incantation of the breast" was recited:

> This is the breast from which Isis suffered in the marsh of Khemmis when she brought Shu and Tefnut into the world. What she did for [her breasts] was to cast a spell with the *iar*-plant, with a pod of the *seneb*-plant, with the part of the rush, with the [fibers of the inner part

This bottle dates from the 18th to 20th Dynasties. Milk from a healthy mother is thought to have been poured in the head and allowed to flow from the open nipples of the breasts into the newborn's mouth. Evidence suggests that watching this process may have stimulated the new mother's milk to begin flowing. Rosicrucian Egyptian Museum, San Jose, California.

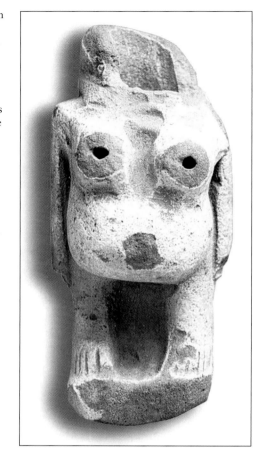

(ib) of the rush], in order to drive away the action of a dead man, or of a dead woman, and so on. Prepare this in the form of a bandage twisted toward the left that shall be set upon [the place of] the action of the dead man or dead woman [with the following words]: "Do not provoke evacuations! Do not make substances that eat [the flesh]! Do not draw blood. Take care so that [malign substances causing] obscurity [blurred vision] to occur in human beings do not occur in [you]." Words to be said over the *iar*-plant, over the part of the *seneb*-plant,

on the bandage twisted to the left, in which seven knots are to be made. [It] shall be knots. Apply [it] to that. (Ebers 811)

In the event of harm to the mother's breasts, application of a poultice containing calamine (a product of oxidized metals often employed today in the treatment of inflammations of mucous membranes and of the skin) was recommended: "Another remedy for a painful breast: calamine: 1; bile of ox: 1; flyspecks: 1; ochre: 1. Make [this] as one thing [that is, a homogeneous mass or smooth mixture]. Smear the breast with [it] for four days in a row" (Ebers 810).[23]

Despite all these precautions, the infant might prove recalcitrant and, by refusing the breast, help to bring about his own demise. In this case medicine once again exploited the resources of magic to persuade him to drink: "Horus will swallow and Seth will chew . . ." (Ramesseum III, B, 10–11). Certain formulas actually sought to "quench the thirst of an infant":

> Your hunger is taken away by . . . , your thirst is [taken away] by Ageb-Ur up into the sky. O bird [*pakh*], your thirst is in my fist, your hunger is in my claw . . . The cow Hesat [puts?] its teat in your mouth. Your mouth is like the mouth of the bird [*khabesu*] on the breath [that goes out from the body] of Osiris. You will not eat your hunger, you will not drink [your thirst] . . . your gullet will not become unfeeling. May a man say this formula over a flat cake [?] of earth, placed on a bandage of linen . . . put in the form of [?]. (Ramesseum III, B, 14–17).

As a last resort, newborns deprived of mother's milk and of the services of a wet nurse were fed cow's milk.[24] Images of royal male infants sucking from the udders of the divine cow of Hathor suggest that hollow cows' horns or anthropomorphic vases in the shape of a kneeling woman or goddess, with a child on her lap, were filled with milk to serve as artificial nipples.[25]

6 Childhood and Adolescence

The attentions enjoyed by the newborn infant did not diminish with time. Once weaned from its mother's breast, the child remained the object of constant care: "The love of children is one of the characteristic traits of the Egyptians and they let no occasion pass them by for lavishing it, sometimes even with a certain ostentation one might say." The long period of breastfeeding conferred a degree of protection against microbial digestive disorders that their ample diet, described by Diodorus, was intended to preserve after weaning:

> They feed their children in a sort of happy-go-lucky fashion that in its expansiveness quite surpasses belief; for they serve them with stews made of any stuff that is ready to hand and cheap, and give them such stalks of the *byblos* plant as can be roasted in the coals, and the roots and stems of marsh plants, either raw or boiled or baked. And since most of the children are reared without shoes or clothing because of the mildness of the climate of the country, the entire expense incurred by the parents of the child until it comes to maturity is not more than twenty drachmas. These are the leading reasons why Egypt has such a large population.[1]

Childhood
Ailments

Children in ancient Egypt were nonetheless vulnerable to various complaints, which ranged from the ordinary cough to *saa*, a strange illness that is still unidentified today, as well as urinary problems, cutaneous eruptions, and head colds. Though the extant medical papyri mention

A mother generally carried her infant in a pouch fastened around her neck. In this detail of a bas-relief from the 19th Dynasty tomb of Haremheb at Biban el-Muluk, a second child is shown astride the mother's shoulders. Rijksmuseum van Oudheden, Leiden.

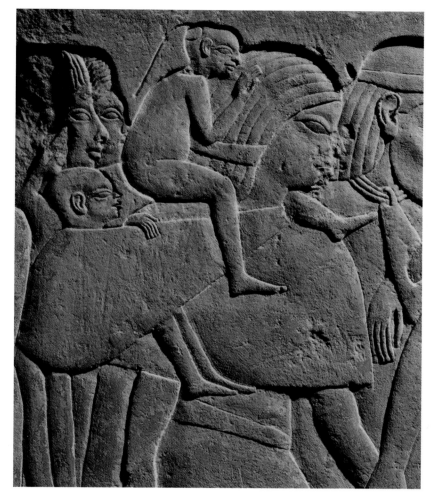

few remedies devised expressly for treating small children, many prescriptions were suitable for young and old alike. Calming certain cries of pain might call for a recipe specifically meant for children, however, such as the one made from a plant called *shepen*—possibly the opium poppy, a renowned sedative and painkiller: "Remedy for relieving much crying *(ashaut):* parts of the *shepen*-plant; flies' excrement that is on the wall. Prepare [this] as one thing, mash, and take for four [consecutive] days. [It] will cease completely. As for 'much crying,' it concerns a child who cries [continually]" (Ebers 782).[2]

Another substance known as *tjehenet,* made from a mixture of faience and an unspecified Nubian gem, was supposed to cure an infantile condition that is still quite common today: "What must be prepared for a child who suffers from wetness: *tjehenet* boiled [and made] in the form of a ball. If the child is already big he will ingest it [as it is]. If he is still in swaddling clothes, it is to be ground up in milk by his nurse, and he will suck on it for four days [in a row]" (Ebers 273).[3] But this is not the only urinary problem noticed in children. Elsewhere in the Ebers papyrus mention is made of an "accumulation of urine" that might be a case of urinary retention: "Another [remedy], so that a child evacuates an accumulation of urine that is inside his belly: a used papyrus [sheet]. Boil [it] in oil and smear his body [with it] until his evacuation is normal" (Ebers 262).

More than the preparation itself, which was applied to the belly of the young patient, it was the mechanical stimulation of the abdominal massage that enabled him to urinate. But treating the child alone was not enough. It was also necessary to care for the mother, who was considered responsible for the urinary troubles of her offspring: "Another [remedy], to make the urine of a child normal: marrow that is in the reed. Grind it in a *khau*-vase of sweet beer, so that it thickens. [It] will be drunk by the woman, and [some] will be given to the child as well in a *henu*-vase" (Ebers 272 bis).

Another concern was the onset of teething. In ancient Egypt, as in our own day, the "tooth fairy" played a role in this, but it was far from being purely symbolic—at least according to Lefebvre, who saw the following recipe as a means of comforting small children when their first teeth penetrated the gums: "The child and [his] mother are to eat a cooked mouse. Its bones are placed around the [child's] neck in a tissue of fine linen [in which] seven knots are tied" (Berlin 3027, verso 8, 2–3).[4]

Mice are everywhere in Egyptian medicine. Whole or in part, they figure in ointments for rheumatic pain and for treatment of the scalp. But this teething remedy seems to have enjoyed particular popularity, for rodent bones have been found in the digestive tracts of several children buried in a cemetery of the Predynastic Period. Curiously, from the sixteenth century until the early twentieth century there was a revival of cures involving mice in the form of decoctions meant to relieve urinary incontinence, dental troubles, and whooping cough.[5]

Otorhinological Disorders

A paragraph in the Ebers papyrus suggests that what modern medicine calls the otorhinolaryngological or ear-nose-throat (ENT) system was similarly conceived by the ancient Egyptians in terms of the seven orifices of the head: nostrils, eyes, ears, and mouth. This passage describes a condition, very similar to what we now call sinusitis, that was treated with a preparation made from milk and gum and accompanied by the following magical incantation:

> Flow out [from the nose], *rech*-exudate, . . . [you] who make painful the seven holes of the head of the servants of Ra and worshippers of Thoth. Behold! I have brought your remedy against you, your potion against you: milk of [a] woman who has borne a male child, fragrant gum. It shall drive you away! It shall put you to flight! It shall put you to flight! It shall drive you away! Go down into the earth, break [yourself] apart, break [yourself] apart. [To be said] four times. Words to be said four times over the milk of [a] woman having borne a male child [and over] fragrant gum. Place [it] in the nose. (Ebers 763)

This same papyrus refers to the common cold, coryza, by a variety of names. Three kinds of exuded substance are mentioned: *khenet,* from the decomposition of a pathogenic substance called *setet;* another called *rech;* and a third called *nia* whose origin has yet to be discovered. For each of these there were medical remedies:

> Another [remedy] to drive out *khenet*-exudate from the nose: galena: 1; rotten wood: 1; dry frankincense: 1; honey: 1; paint the eye with [it] for four days [in a row]. Do [it]! You will see [the result]! It is truly excellent!
>
> Remedy for the *rech*-exudate: date wine. Fill up the opening [of the nose].
>
> Another [remedy] to drive out the *nia*-exudate from the nose: *niaia*-plant. Crush [this] with dates and apply to the nose. (Ebers 418, 761, 762)

Still more interestingly, the case of a child complaining of earache—very probably due to infection (otitis media)—furnishes evidence of a true therapeutic attitude in dealing with the stages in the development of the condition that lend themselves to diagnosis (Berlin 200–204). The first symptoms, characterized by a "sensation of heaviness of the ear," were treated by a method that combines the antiseptic properties of turpentine with the anti-inflammatory action of celery. The insistent pain of the second phase of otitis media was relieved with a preparation made from cumin, a spice having antiseptic and anti-inflammatory effect: "[. . .]: pyrethrum seeds: 1/64; cumin: 1/64; *peret-sheny*-fruit: 1/64; seed of *aru*-tree: 1/8; *ankh-imy*-plant: 1/4; melilot: 1/32; acacia leaves: 1/32; [. . .] of *djai*: 1/64; honey: 1/8; sweet beer: 15 *ro*. Reduce to ashes. [This] to be drunk by the man [or child]" (Berlin 204).

Other preparations described elsewhere in the medical corpus were aimed at treating the purulent discharge from the ear that characterizes the third phase, serous otitis media. In the absence of complicating factors, the ear was sometimes fumigated with crocodile droppings, frogs' eggs, and tortoise shell, or, in the case of inflammation of the outer ear, by "a cold treatment [for] it must not be hot. If a vessel trembles, you must prepare for it: chip *(shepa)* of malachite" (Ebers 766).

Another passage appears to refer to an ear plugged up with wax: "If [the opening of the ear] is oily [serous] on account of that, you must prepare for it the [following] treatment, which is meant to dry out a wound: head of rodent; gall bladder of goat; shell of tortoise; fleawort. Sprinkle [the ear] with that very often" (Ebers 766).

If medicine failed, or if the child was not healed by other means, the consequences could be dramatic, not only physiologically but socially as well. Jacques Willemot has argued that children incapable of speaking by the age of three (almost certainly as a result of deafness) were considered to be possessed, and for this reason were drowned in the Nile, while older deaf persons were relegated to the ranks of slaves. The latter claim is difficult to prove, even if it is probable that such people were treated as simple animals, on the same level as an anencephalic child.[6]

Bronchopulmonary Ailments   The Egyptians grouped all bronchopulmonary ailments under the generic term "cough" *(seryt)*, which on Bardinet's reading they interpreted as "jolts due to secretions," that is, expectoration. But there were various ways to treat this symptom—forty ways, to be precise. This is the total number of therapeutic preparations found in the Ebers, Berlin, and Hearst papyri, some of which were intended for both children and adults.

The beneficial properties of some of the ingredients that figure in these medicines are still recognized today: honey, a famously soothing remedy, is mentioned twelve times; also cream, milk, and a variety of sweet products such as carob (the edible pulp of the pods of the carob tree) and date pulp, which calm irritation, as well as melilot (also called sweet clover), a herbaceous plant with very fragrant flowers that contain coumarin, an antitussive, antispasmodic, and diuretic substance. More surprisingly, colocynth, generally known for its purgative properties, is sometimes found in these remedies. Its use suggests that the physician sought to expel illness from the body if treatment did not make it disappear.[7]

To relieve chronic coughing Dioscorides prescribed cumin in combination with a high-calorie diet, a regime still recommended today for severe pulmonary infections. But he also laid special emphasis on the value of medicaments that the patient inhaled.[8] Indeed the Egyptians were largely responsible for establishing the benefits of this treatment, whose first mention in the history of medicine occurs in the Ebers papyrus: "You shall take seven stones, and you shall heat them in a fire. You shall take one of these stones and place some of the medication on top of it. You shall cover it with a new pot, whose bottom has been perforated, and you shall put a reed stalk in the hole. You shall place your mouth over the opening of this stalk in order to be able to inhale the vapor coming out of it" (Ebers 325).

Inhalation therapy was widely adopted by the other medical traditions of antiquity for its therapeutic and hygienic effects. Fumigation—the use of smoke or vapor as a disinfectant or to destroy pests—was commonly employed as well, as part of a program of public hygiene.[9] Medicines were not prescribed for longer than four days, perhaps a symbolic period of time given that the number four was considered, particularly during the Old Kingdom, to have magical and beneficial value.

Malevolent Substances and Demons

Translating the names for disease found in the medical papyri into modern terms is sometimes a puzzling business. The Hearst papyrus, for example, mentions what appears to be an infantile disease, marked by a violent cutaneous eruption and attributed to the action of a mysterious substance known as *temiet:* "Remedy for driving out the *temiet*-substance: charcoal; *shenef(et)*-plant, liquid dregs; flour [. . .] [left on] the [threshing] floor [of wheat]; *didi*-mineral; emmer; *sherypededu*-plant; sea salt. Cook [this]. Dress with it" (Hearst 168). And: "Another [remedy]: fruit of the ricinus [castor-oil] plant; seeds of *nechau*-plant; dates; peas; pyrethrum seed; *ta*-liquid from the tanner [a bleach used in tanning]; honey. To be administered as before" (Hearst 169).

A magical spell contained in section B of the "Book of Protection for Mother and Child," as Papyrus Berlin 3027 is also known, gives some insight into the nature of this dreadful substance: "Another [formula]: Drain off! [You] *temiet*-substance, which shatters the bones [. . .], which enters into the vessels *(metu)*." And in the London papyrus one finds this related spell:

> Incantation for the *temiet*-substance. Heat that comes out of Busiris [. . .] [?]. Isis is in tears, having worshipped the skin of Horus [which is] the skin of such a son of such a [woman]. O ram that descends from heaven at the call of Isis [?]. Ra has spoken [?]. Osiris has spoken [?]. May the flood spray the skin of such a son of such a [woman]. Drain off, heat! Osiris has spoken: he has heard the message [of Ra] and the earth rejoices. Ra is in the temple [. . .] [?]
>
> Words to be spoken four times over: honey; *pa-pur*-liquid; *saur*-resin; flour of [. . .] [left on] the [threshing] floor [of the wheat]. (London 6)

Elsewhere this substance is associated with a demon called a *nesiet.* Another long spell in the London papyrus made it possible to struggle against these combined scourges, whose severity, construed as the expression of divine punishment, warranted recourse to the magic of the gods:

> Another [incantation to drive out] the *nesiet*-demon and the *temiet*-substance that Isis made for her father, in accordance with what was made for him [. . .].
>
> By the Great Ennead that faced those assembled in the chapel on the day when [Isis] paid tribute,

The night when Osiris opened his mouth to speak before the pure
Place, saying:
My son Horus shall avenge me!
And this is why his son Horus shall avenge him. (London 25)

Pascal Hennequin has made the intriguing suggestion that the *nesiet*-demon may be associated with convulsions that accompany nervous disorder in children. If so, the condition uniting the *temiet*-substance and the *nesiet*-demon might well be measles, which combines dermatological symptoms with remarkable neurological disturbances.[10]

The baa *Disease*

Precise hypotheses are not always possible, however. Unlike the condition caused by the *temiet*-substance, the *baa* disease, repeatedly mentioned in texts concerning childhood maladies, remains thoroughly mysterious. A corrupt passage in Ramesseum III (B, 20–23) appears to counsel the use of spells and amulets to ward it off: "To drive out the *baa*: to say as a magical formula [. . .] acacia. Turn [it] to the left and put around the neck of the child. This is a way of driving out the *baa*." Papyrus Berlin 3027 (7, 1–3) recommends the following remedy: "To repel the *baa*: parts of the sycamore: fresh dates; part of the ricinus [castor-oil] plant; hemp; fibrous wad [made from the filaments] of the *debiet*-plant; *mesta*-liquid. [This] to be drunk by the woman."

A closer look at the textual evidence supplies a few clues. We know that the mother was thought to be the healthy carrier of the *baa*-substance, which was transmitted to the child through her milk. Additionally, the remedy was administered to the mother in order to treat the child, as if her milk were equally capable of transmitting poison and antidotes. During the process of contamination the *baa* spread throughout the child's body, destroying his internal organs. So grave was this illness that incantations invoking Isis herself failed to cure him. It fell to the arts of magic, then, to repulse the *baa* and push it back into the swallow, the bird whose form Isis had assumed when the body of Osiris was shut up in its coffin (Ramesseum III, B, 23–24).

A number of scholars have sought to identify this obscure malady, so far without success. Warren R. Dawson thought it might be a diet-related condition; Hermann Grapow suggested a disease contracted by the mother, who infected her child in turn. Thierry Bardinet, for his part, sees it as the result of an airborne pathogen transmitted by breast-feeding.[11] A more precise identification may one day be possible. For the moment, however, we can say only that the Egyptians held this invisible agent responsible for several different childhood illnesses, which they grouped together under the same term because of their common origin.

Adolescence

No text or scene of daily life in ancient Egypt that has come down to us portrays the physiological changes of adolescence. Only the drawing of a scarab (dung) beetle, symbol of Khepri (god of the dawn and, more generally, of transformation), discreetly placed next to a figure above a cartouche, distinguishes adolescents from other figures on the walls of temples and tombs. We do know that, for a boy, the end of childhood was marked by rites of passage to adulthood: his long hair was cut and he was presented with a loincloth and circumcised.

Circumcision and the Onset of Menstruation

Circumcision was undergone by young men at the age of sixteen or seventeen. Although the surviving medical papyri do not mention this procedure, there is some evidence that Egyptians performed circumcisions as early as the third millennium B.C.[12] The hieroglyphic sign for the phallus (translated, depending on the context, as "phallus," "male," or the verbal phrase "to copulate" or "to urinate") depicts this organ without a foreskin. It cannot be concluded, however, that this custom was everywhere and always observed, for uncircumcised mummies dating from the New Kingdom have been found. The fact that Ahmose I, a pharaoh of the 18th Dynasty, was not circumcised, though his father and his brothers were, has aroused considerable speculation among Egyptologists. Arnauld Bellouard has suggested that Ahmose's fragile constitution may have been due to a generalized form of osteoarthritis, principally affecting his knees, but perhaps also evidence of hemophilia. If so, circumcision would have been a risky procedure.[13]

The cultural significance of circumcision among the Egyptians remains unclear as well. Some authorities, pointing to a passage in the *Book of the Dead,* maintain that it was a religious ritual recalling the example of the sun god: "Blood fell from the phallus of Ra after he had finished cutting himself." Other authors have seen it as a hygienic mea-

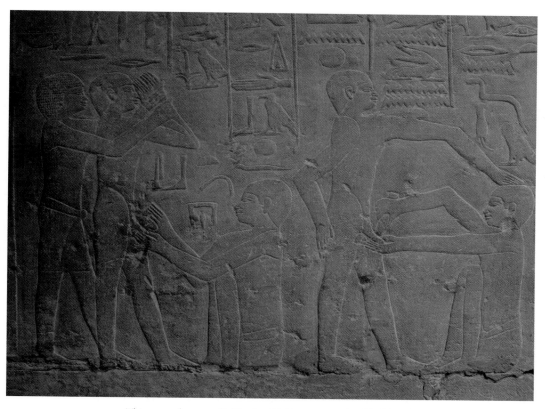

This scene from a relief in the 6th Dynasty tomb of Ankhmahor at Saqqara has usually been interpreted as a ritual circumcision performed by a *hemka*-priest on a young boy. Recent scholarship suggests that instead it may depict an initiation rite for *hemka*-priests, in which the pubis of the novice is shaved.

sure. Herodotus, referring to priests, says: "They practice circumcision for cleanliness' sake, preferring to be clean rather than comely."[14]

A bas-relief from the 6th Dynasty, found on a wall of the *mastaba*-tomb of Ankhmahor at Saqqara, depicts the two stages of the procedure. The first panel shows a young man standing in front of a squatting figure who appears to be applying a preparation of some sort. In the inscription that accompanies this scene the subject says, "Rub [it] well in order that [it] may be effective," to which the surgeon responds,

"[I] will make it comfortable"—suggesting the use of a form of anesthesia, very possibly "Memphis stone." An assistant grips the young man's arms from behind, holding his hands in front of his eyes. The surgeon says to the assistant: "Hold him fast! Do not let him fall [if he faints]." The second panel shows the surgeon taking hold of the young man's phallus and making the circumcision with obsidian (or, as Herodotus calls it in another context, a sharp knife of Ethiopian stone).[15]

With regard to rites of passage for young girls on attaining the age of womanhood, by contrast, our sources are silent. While no medical document refers to the onset of menstruation, the Ebers papyrus does mention a treatment to be administered after several years of amenorrhea:

> If you examine a woman who has spent many years without her menstruation coming. She spits out something like *hebeb*-liquid. Her belly is like the inside of a body that is on fire. It ceases when she has vomited.
>
> Then you shall say concerning it/her: it is a raising up of blood in her uterus because it has cast a spell upon her. You shall prepare for it: juniper berries: 1/32; cumin: 1/64; turpentine: 1/64; rhizome of the rush nut: 1/16. You shall take cow's milk, 80 *ro*, heated with [ox] bone marrow. Place [the mixture] in this milk. To be drunk for four days [in a row]. (Ebers 833)

Heartache and Lovesickness

The physiological changes of adolescence were accompanied by other disturbances. Like our own children, young people in ancient Egypt felt the first flutterings of love and suffered the pain of longing and rejection. Then, as now, girls sought to make themselves desired by boys who they hoped might one day become their husbands. Consider the testimony of one young man:

> My beloved knows how to lasso [a steer]
> Without having to count the herd.
> With her hair she throws her net around me,
> With her eyes she takes me prisoner,
> With her finery she overcomes me,
> With her tongue she marks me with a branding iron.

Young women, too, were known to express their feelings for their beloved:

When I take him in my arms
And when his arms wrap themselves around me,
It is like [being] in the land of Punt,
It is as though [my] body were immersed in a fragrant oil.
When I embrace him
And when his lips are parted
I feel drunk
Without having had any beer to drink.[16]

And then, as now, amorous passion was apt to give way to profound melancholy. In Papyrus Chester Beatty I, we encounter a young man who seems to have experienced the suffering brought on by lovesickness as an unknown and incurable disease:

If the master-physicians come to me, my heart is immune to their remedy.
Exorcists? No comfort can be had from them [for] my illness has not been diagnosed.
But being able to say: here she is—that is what [will] revive me.
My salvation [will be] that she comes in here.
I will see her and I will be cured.
She will open her eyes and my legs will be young again.
She will speak to me and I will be strong [again].
I will embrace her and she will cast my illness aside.[17]

Another kind of illness, jealousy, was experienced by women who found themselves confronted with a rival. In this case the jealous lover might resort to magic to make the hair of a detested woman fall out, smearing her rival's head with "cooked *anart*-worm, boiled in grease." The equally unappetizing antidote to this was made from "hippopotamus shank and tortoise shell" (Ebers 474, 476).

Youthful Excess   We should not be surprised to learn that lovesick youths in pharaonic times drowned their sorrows in alcohol. In addition to water from the Nile, the Egyptians consumed great quantities of milk—from goats, sheep, and cows—and beer made from cereals (chiefly barley, but also summer wheat). Wine was a true luxury item, which only the wealthiest could afford to drink regularly. During the Old Kingdom there were six kinds of wine—among them white, red, and black, and a vintage from

Lower Egypt—as well as another alcoholic beverage, *shedeh,* that is cited in a number of texts.[18] Adolescents drank in public taverns, often to excess. The following tirade has been preserved of a mother sharply rebuking her son for his dissolute ways:

I am told that you neglect the practice of writing
And that you give yourself over to a life of pleasure.
You go from tavern to tavern,
Beer takes away your respect for others,
You lead your spirit astray.
You are like a broken rudder
That is good for nothing.
You are like a chapel without a god,
Like a home without bread.
You were seen trying to jump over a wall.
People flee from [your] dangerous blows.
Ah! If [only] you understood that wine
Is an abomination.
You would curse sweet wine,
You would not think of beer,
[You] would forget wine from other lands.[19]

Many mothers would undoubtedly have preferred that their sons follow the teaching of the sage Any, who urged moderation in the consumption of alcohol: "Do not go too far in drinking a large pitcher of beer! When you speak, incomprehensible words come out of your mouth. You fall down, you break your limbs, and no one lends you a hand. Your drinking companions get up and say: Let's rid ourselves of this drunkard! When one comes to look for you and ask your advice, you are found lying on the ground and you are like a small child."[20] Nor were young women innocent of such unseemly behavior. In the tomb of a high official from the 18th Dynasty named Pahery, at Elkab, a woman is shown clamoring for refreshment: "Give me eighteen cups of wine. Do you not see that I wish to make myself drunk? My insides are dry like straw."[21]

But beware the morning after! The Insinger papyrus contains this familiar admonition: "He who has too much wine will be filled up, a hangover will keep him in bed."[22]

7 Old Age and Deformities

No less than ourselves today the Egyptians sought to square the circle, looking to find ways to retain their faculties in old age. At the end of a full life a person might hope to attain the glorious age of 110 years. The significance of this canonical figure, frequently cited in the texts that have come down to us, seems to have been primarily symbolic and closely associated with the notion of wisdom. Wishes for prosperity and long life were commonly expressed with reference to it. Thus we read in a letter addressed to the sage Amenemope by one of his disciples: "May [safe passage to] Amenti be granted to you, without having experienced [the miseries of] old age, without having been ill. May you finish out 110 years on earth, your limbs remaining vigorous, since it is in this way that a blessed man such as yourself must be rewarded by his god."[1]

Certain eminent figures, among them the celebrated magus Djedi ("a simple individual of 110 years"), are recorded as having attained this age. Others came close, such as Pepy III and, most famously of all, Rameses II, an illustrious warrior who lived to be at least 80, apparently without requiring any special care, having produced 96 sons and 60 daughters by 200 wives. Nebenteru, high priest of the 21st Dynasty, is said to have lived to be almost 100. An epitaph engraved on his statue reads: "I passed my life in joy, without either worry or illness [. . .] and thus I exceeded the years of each one of my contemporaries. Try and make sure such a thing happens to you."[2]

Such luck was rare. Indeed, to judge from the persistence of connective cartilage observed in corpses from the pharaonic period, very few people seem to have lived beyond what we now consider middle age.

Rates of infant mortality, impossible to estimate with certainty but surely quite high, suggest that average life expectancy was between thirty and thirty-five years. This result is corroborated by an analysis of 709 adult skulls in the collection of the Museo Egizio in Turin, which placed the average age of death at about thirty years during the Predynastic Period and at thirty-six during the Dynastic Period.[3] In all likelihood the very small number of cancers found is to be attributed to low life expectancy rather than to dietary or genetic factors: malignant tumors did not have enough time to develop.

The Indignities of Growing Old

The ravages of old age were no less dreaded in ancient Egypt than they are today. Mute testimony to this apprehension may be found in the hieroglyphic character for "old man," a bent-over figure leaning on a staff for support. Ptahhotep, in his maxims, describes the decrepitude that overtook him late in life:

> Sovereign, my lord, great age is here, old age has descended upon me; languor has come, the weakness of infancy returns, so that he who has once again become an infant continually sleeps. The arms are weak, the legs have given up obeying the heart, which has become tired. The mouth is silent, it can no longer speak; the eyes are weak, the ears are deaf; the nose is stuffed up, it can no longer breathe. All sense of taste has gone away. The mind is forgetful, it cannot remember yesterday. The bones hurt in old age; both getting up and sitting down are difficult. What was good has become bad. What old age does to men is evil in every way.

Not even the gods were protected against physical decline: "Ra appears every day at the head of the crew of the solar bark and assumes the throne of the double horizon. Age makes his mouth tremble and his spittle drips onto the ground."[4]

From the most ancient times, then, there has been a desire to disguise or eliminate the signs of degeneration. Thus, for example, in the magical part of the Edwin Smith papyrus (verso 21) we find a recipe for "transforming an old man into a young man." The Ebers papyrus mentions a variety of cosmetic preparations designed "to transform the skin," "to open up the outer flesh," "to stretch the face," "to drive away wrinkles from the face" (Ebers 714, 713, 716). One such remedy promises to "beautify the skin" by giving it a fashionable pallor: "Another [remedy] to beautify the skin: powdered alabaster, 1; powdered natron, 1; sea salt, 1; honey, 1. Mix [this] together as one thing with the honey. Smear the skin with [it]" (Ebers 715).

As they aged the Egyptians were vulnerable to much more serious dermatological problems. Although the skin is often missing, and despite the tinting and hardening of the skin caused by embalming, macroscopic examination of mummies has made it possible to diagnose such disorders. Despite the difficulties associated with visual inspection of cutaneous lesions, it remains a valuable source of information, compensating for the silence of the papyri on this point—a silence that is complete except for the "substances that eat [away at]" (Ebers 589) and possible itches (Ebers 591, 615). The existence of senile acne, for example, is attested by the blackheads noted on certain mummies of old men (the forehead of Rameses II himself appears to have been dotted with small brownish-red tumors). Attempts to remove these unsightly marks were made even after death. Thus, in the case of a priestess of Amun who lived during the 21st Dynasty, embalmers tried to conceal sores on the buttocks and the back (no doubt caused by a prolonged period of confinement to bed prior to death) with pieces of gazelle hide.[5]

Advancing age also took its toll on the scalp, on which great care was lavished by both men and women earlier in life. Women often wore their hair long and curled and left their children's wavy locks uncut. Priests shaved their heads and bodies. Herodotus notes the effectiveness of shaving the head to protect against hair loss: "The Egyptians shave their heads from childhood, and the bone thickens from exposure to the sun. This is also the reason why they do not grow bald; for nowhere can one see so few bald heads as in Egypt."[6]

Despite these precautions baldness sometimes occurred late in life, as the examination of mummies confirms. At the time of his death Rameses II still had relatively thick hair at his temples and on the back of his head,[7] whereas Amenhotep III and Sety I had become nearly bald. Nor were women spared this embarrassment. Queen Nefertari, wife of Rameses II, who suffered from alopecia, wore a wig to cover her bare skull. Fear of baldness led the Egyptians to concoct various recipes for stimulating lost hair to grow back, each one stranger than the last: "An-

Baldness was reputed to be exceptionally rare among the ancient Egyptians. Examination of the mummy of Rameses II, who is shown here as a youthful hunter with a long, braided side lock, has revealed that he retained much of his hair in old age. Limestone bas-relief now in the Louvre.

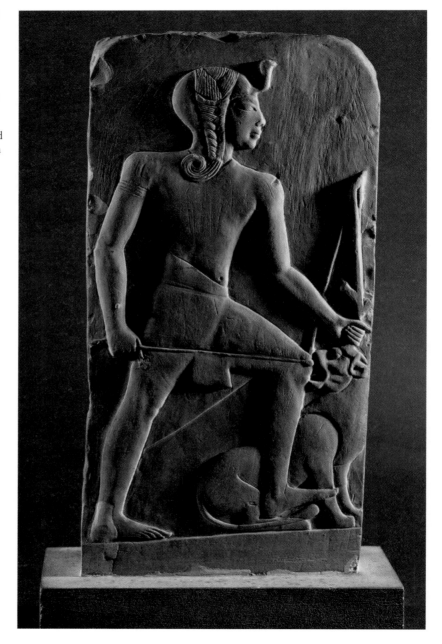

other [remedy] to cause hair to grow on a bald person: fat [*adj*] of lion, 1; fat of hippopotamus, 1; fat of crocodile, 1; fat of cat, 1; fat of snake, 1; fat of ibex, 1. Make as one thing. Smear the head of the bald person with [it]" (Ebers 465).[8] Here we find a good example of the principle of analogy, well known among magicians, according to which fresh vitality could be gained from contact with parts of certain animals, in particular the lion with its noble mane. Other remedies call for a "donkey's hoof," "flyspecks," and "[blood of] dogs' vulvas" (Ebers 468, 774, 460).

Older persons who worried about their appearance could also hope to arrest the graying of their hair with an unusual lotion: "Another [remedy] for truly driving away the substance that ravages [the hair] and to care for the hair: blood of black ox. Place [this] in fat/oil *(merhet)*. Smear [the hair] with [it]" (Ebers 459).

Rheumatism and Failing Eyesight

The radiological study of mummies has deepened our understanding of various rheumatic conditions from which the ancient Egyptians suffered. Arthritis has been observed in many pharaohs: spinal arthritis in Amenhotep I, cervical in Merenptah. X-rays of Rameses II have made it possible to propose a more complete diagnosis involving erosion of the sacroiliac joints in the lumbar region of the spine and the pelvis, a paradoxical enlargement of the intervertebral spaces, and general calcification of the anterior longitudinal ligament.[9] Twenty prescriptions contained in the Ramesseum and Ebers papyri concern rheumatic conditions. Thus one finds remedies for "relaxing the juncture between two parts of the body," "relaxing a stiff part," "healing a bone anywhere in the body of a man," or "loosening up stiff parts anywhere in the body" (Ebers 656, 658, 654, 670, 675). Derived in the main from animal and vegetable fats, these soothing balms and ointments incorporated bone marrow, flour, natron, ox's spleen, gum, incense, celery, onions, cumin, juniper, acacia juice—and even mud (Ebers 656).

Motor function is not the only faculty that deteriorates with age: sight is also affected. In ancient Egypt, heat, dust, insects, and poor hygiene were all apt to favor ocular disease. In this regard preservation of corpses does not help us make retrospective diagnoses, for the process of mummification was always accompanied by dehydration and retraction of the eyeballs. What information we have comes from the

Ebers and Kahun papyri, which mention among other things a probable xanthelasma (fatty yellow plaque on the eyelid), described as "grease that is in the eyes," as well as remedies intended to drive out evil substances causing "cloudiness in an eye" and "weakness of sight" (Ebers 354, 339, 340, 415).[10]

Cataracts, which often develop with age, seem to be referred to in a passage in Ebers, if Paul Ghalioungui is right, by the phrase "rise of water"—an expression that was later to be encountered with the Greeks *(hypochysis)* and the Romans *(suffusio)*.[11] Some commentators have seen evidence of cataracts in at least one image of Nefertiti, queen of Akhenaten, whose right eye is blank on a magnificent limestone bust that has come down to us.[12] But even if she actually did suffer from cataracts, we are ignorant as to the Egyptians' methods of treatment. We do not know whether they treated cataracts with surgery, for example. A neighboring people, the Akkadians of Mesopotamia, are known to have used a technique called "lowering," which consisted in moving the lens of the eye downward with a needle until the patient could see again.[13] But this subject remains controversial. Our only source for the surgical treatment of cataracts in ancient Egypt is the Stoic philosopher Chryssipus, writing in the third century B.C., who maintained that it was common. The Greek surgeon Antyllus of Alexandria is said to have operated on cataracts in the second century A.D.

Cardiovascular Disorders

Like skin and bones, internal organs wear out over time, and the risk of cardiovascular problems increases with age. Though they did not specify the age of their patients, Egyptian physicians left a detailed study of these disorders in the "Book of the Heart," a section of the Ebers papyrus (854–855z) that reveals an impressive grasp of cardiovascular function. The descriptions of several pathologies contained in this papyrus—cardiac insufficiency and dysrhythmia, infarction of the myocardium, arterial aneurysm—are remarkably perceptive.[14]

The analysis of cardiac insufficiency, and of its hepatic consequences, suggests that the Egyptians understood the link between the liver and the circulation of blood. In the Ebers papyrus (854I) we find explicit reference to the "four vessels *(metu)* [that] go to the liver; they give it liquids and breath [that is, dynamic current]." Cardiac insufficiency, designated by the term *khasef* ("weakness that exists in the heart"), was said to have repercussions "as far as the lungs and the liver" and to produce a state of cardiogenic shock in which the patient "becomes deaf" and his pulse is indiscernible, the vessels having "sunk" and the extremities grown cold "after their heat [has gone away]" (Ebers 855d). In extremely serious cases, the "inside *(ib)* weakens": arterial tension—the pressure of blood within the arteries—falls drastically, and the pulse, now too rapid, becomes thready. In addition to these symptoms there are disturbing neurological signs of reduced blood flow to the brain, manifested by torpor and lethargy, which the papyrus describes thus: "The heart *(haty)* no longer speaks or the vessels of the heart *(haty)* are dumb, giving no sign under the hands [of the doctor]" (Ebers 855e).[15]

With regard to disruption of the cardiac rhythm, Egyptian physicians seem to have recognized the relationship between good health and the fixed and stable localization of the heart. Several glosses of the papyrus affirm that abnormal cardiac position is synonymous with disease, and forecast an attack against the entire body when this organ "moves away from its place." The gloss at Ebers 855p is an example: "As to 'the heart *(haty)* is in its place,' this means that the mass of the heart is on the left side of the man and that it can neither go up or down because it is fixed in its place." And the Louvre papyrus includes this instruction: "Do so that my inside *(ib)* is fixed in its proper place" (no. 3279, I, 12).

In what is called the "dance of the heart *(haty),*" the patient's heart is observed to "move away from the left breast"—a displacement of the apex that today is diagnosed in cases of simple tachycardia or arrhythmia due to an increase in cardiac volume (Ebers 855n).[16] But when "the heart *(haty)* of the man does not beat much" and "moves downward a bit"—when, in other words, a lessening of cardiac pulsation causes the heart to move away from its place, the hour is late in the eyes of the Egyptian physician: "The [bodily] alteration of the man will spread" (Ebers 855q).

Grave concern was also warranted by the appearance of a series of pains whose description suggests to the modern mind an attack of angina pectoris, or even myocardial infarction. A patient "who suffers at the entrance to the inside *(ib),* when he has pains in his arm, his breast, and the side of his stomach *(ro-ib)*" is said to have little chance of recovering: "Death is approaching" (Ebers 191).[17]

More generally, angiological disorders of the circulatory system were well known to the physicians of pharaonic Egypt, who described varicose veins as well as the dreaded arterial aneurysm (Ebers 872–873).[18] Clinical analysis had brought out the distinctively pulsating and expansive character of the latter condition. Thus a paragraph in Ebers begins: "If you examine a swelling of the vessels in any part of a man and you find it round, and growing beneath your hands with each beat" (872). The author goes on to name the cause of this arterial dysfunction ("It is the vessels that produce it; it is due to an injury to the vessels") and to direct that it be treated by the *sa hemem*—a specialist in cautery, which in this case involved a metallic instrument or, as Leca has suggested, a burning reed.[19]

Elsewhere the Ebers papyrus gives a precise account of an acute pulmonary edema. "All the parts of the body are weak," it declares, noting that the condition is accompanied by plentiful expectoration of "[excessive] saliva" and a sensation of being smothered that is likened to a "flooding of the inside *(ib)*" (gloss 855b). With regard to other vital organs, however, the knowledge of the ancient Egyptians was rather less complete. They were unaware, for example, of the function of the kidneys, which embalmers left in place in the abdominal cavity. The study of kidneys in mummies has revealed a higher incidence of parenchymal than anatomical lesions. In view of the apparent rarity of kidney stones, it may be supposed that the disorders mentioned in the Ebers papyrus arose from the retention of urine in the bladder (261–263, 270, 271, 283). In order to "make [micturition] normal" it was therefore necessary to assist the passing of urinary stones (263). Evidently a remedy was administered (perhaps against cystitis or some prostate disorder, as Nunn has suggested), with the purpose of eliminating "an obstruction of burning substances in the bladder, when the man suffers retention *(hedbu)* of urine" (265).[20]

Parkinson's Disease and Senile Dementia The deterioration of mental faculties is one of the most painful trials of old age. A passage in the Ebers papyrus ascribes the loss of higher functions to the destructive effect of a morbid breath that spreads through the inside *(ib)*: "As for the fact that the inside *(ib)* perishes and [as for] the loss of memory: it is a breath peculiar to the activity of the lector priest that causes this. When it repeatedly enters the trachea-lung [=

windpipe?], the inside *(ib)* becomes injured by it" (855u). Elsewhere the action of this morbid breath is said to alter the vessels, causing what may well in fact be vascular dementia (855h).[21]

More particularly, some modern readers of the "Book of the *Wekhedu*" (Ebers 856a–h, Berlin 163a–h) have claimed to recognize in the description of disordered function in the upper limbs (as in Ebers 856f: "If he suffers in his shoulder and his fingers tremble") the early signs of Parkinson's disease, a condition that initially manifests itself in unilateral trembling confined mainly to the distal extremities of these limbs.[22] To the ancient Egyptian mind, responsibility for these disorders lay chiefly with a kind of pathogenic entity called *setet* that traveled through the vessels up into the arms: "Another [remedy] for driving out [the substances that cause] trembling in the fingers"; "Another [remedy] for driving out the substances *(daut)* found in any part of the body of a man" (Ebers 623, 625).

The Status of the Handicapped

Congenital malformations typically manifest themselves in infancy. What was the reaction of parents and family on discovering deformity in a newborn child? Opinions are divided. Christiane Desroches-Noblecourt has argued that the presence of a malformation or infirmity from the first years of life was considered a mark of divine grace and inspired respect, noting the testimony of Diodorus with regard to the obligation of parents to keep all children that were born to them. According to Guillemette Andreu, however, "handicapped, malformed children were abandoned; considered to have been rejected by the gods, these abnormal beings were compared to crooked timber from which nothing could be made."[23]

Hunchbacks and Dwarves

The principal evidence favoring Andreu's view derives from the anencephalic mummy of an abandoned child discovered in 1823 by Giuseppe Passalacqua in a tomb at Thebes that also contained mummified monkeys, likewise abandoned. On the other hand, a considerable number of hunchbacked children were evidently allowed to grow to maturity. There are many surviving representations of this osseous deformation, including a Predynastic statuette now in the collection of the

Brussels Museum that shows a man suffering from a high kypho-scoliosis with a carinate thorax. One thinks also of the hunchbacked gardener memorialized by a mural in the tomb of Ipy at Thebes, whose likeness is conserved today at the Metropolitan Museum of Art in New York, and the harpist depicted on an ostracon found at Deir el-Bahri, now at the Metropolitan as well, whose kyphosis was no doubt a consequence of his professional activity. Mummies confirm the presence of osseous tumors. Elliot Smith and Warren Dawson found three osteo-sarcomas—bone cancers—in mummies of the 5th Dynasty, two in the upper part of the humerus and one in the femur. Rarer diseases of the skeleton have also been reported, such as the one exhibited by a child of the 12th Dynasty, suffering from a case of osteogenesis imperfecta (Lobstein's disease, or "brittle bones").[24]

Evidence of another deformity, dwarfism, is found in artistic representations—bas-reliefs and statues—rather than in the medical papyri, which contain no unambiguous descriptions of the underlying metabolic and endocrinal disorders. We know that people with achondroplastic dwarfism *(nemu)* were assigned quite specific responsibilities, acting as custodians of the wardrobe in noble families and as supervisors of the work of goldsmiths. Beginning in the Middle Kingdom they seem to have combined these activities with the role of court jester. They were well integrated into Egyptian society and sometimes occupied enviable positions. One statue now in the Louvre (no. 160) shows Seneb, a funerary priest of the tomb of a great lord of the 5th Dynasty, seated next to his wife and another dwarf.[25]

A final remarkable deformity can very probably be explained as a consequence of poliomyelitis. On a funerary stele dating from about 1450 B.C., during the 18th dynasty, the Syrian doorkeeper Roma is shown making an offering to the goddess Astarte in the company of his wife and son. Under his arm he holds a long staff, no doubt used as a crutch to compensate for the weakness of his atrophied leg and the equinus deformity of the foot, both almost surely due to polio. Another case of polio has been suspected in the 18th Dynasty pharaoh Smenkhkara. The mummy of the pharaoh Saptah, who was about twenty-five when he died, may present another case. His clubbed left foot and shortened leg, compensated for by a hyperextension of the

The "Polio stele." The withered leg and foot of the man identified on this 18th Dynasty limestone stele as "Roma the doorkeeper" have long been attributed to poliomyelitis. Limestone with original paintwork dating to the reign of Amenhotep III. Provenance unknown; acquired in Egypt in the 1890s. Glyptotek Museum, Copenhagen.

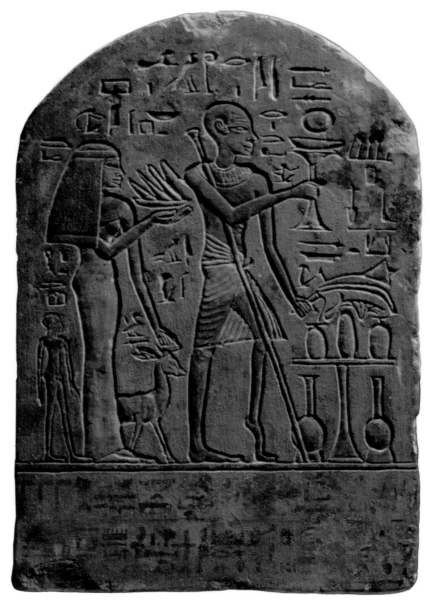

ankle and foot, would seem to suggest the effects of poliomyelitis, but the possibility of a congenital malformation cannot be ruled out.[26]

Illustrious Cases A number of kings and queens are known to have exhibited these deformities. Representations of two of them, in particular, have given rise to extensive commentary and provoked spirited disagreement.

A relief of the queen of Punt in the temple of Hatshepsut at Deir el-Bahri shows a woman of normal height with four adipose folds on her belly and large, flaccid breasts. Her arms and thighs are deformed by enormous rolls of fat that cascade below her knees—without, however, affecting the hands or the feet. Additionally one notes a substantial hyperlordosis (abnormal forward curvature of the spine in the lumbar region), the pelvis being thrust sharply backward. It has been suggested that the queen of Punt may have been a Khoikhoi (Hottentot) from southern Africa. While it is true that we do not know with certainty where the country of Punt was located (Eritrea, Yemen, Sudan, and the southern part of the African continent have all been proposed), Khoikhoi women are small in stature and present a considerable fatty mass in the buttocks. The queen of Punt appears taller than these women, however, and gives the impression of steatopygia only because of her severely swaybacked posture.

Other possible diagnoses for the queen include hypothyroidism with myxedema, and achondroplasia. But the most intriguing possibility is that she was afflicted by Dercum's disease (adiposis dolorosa or lipomatosis neurotica), a condition combining obesity, painful adipose masses in the abdomen and proximal parts of the limbs, and muscular weakness. Moreover, the fatigue from which, on this hypothesis, the queen seems likely to have suffered is suggested by the artist, who has taken care to place a saddled donkey behind her.[27]

Then there is the famously perplexing case of Akhenaten (Amenhotep IV), whose dysmorphism has been a source of great speculation, all the more so because his mummy has not been found. All surviving representations of this pharaoh portray a face with elongated features and a prominent and narrow chin, a long and weak neck, a small chest, a bulging abdomen, an enlarged pelvis, and excessive breast development (gynecomastia). On one statue that shows him naked the genitals are not visible. This asexual depiction of Akhenaten has led some scholars

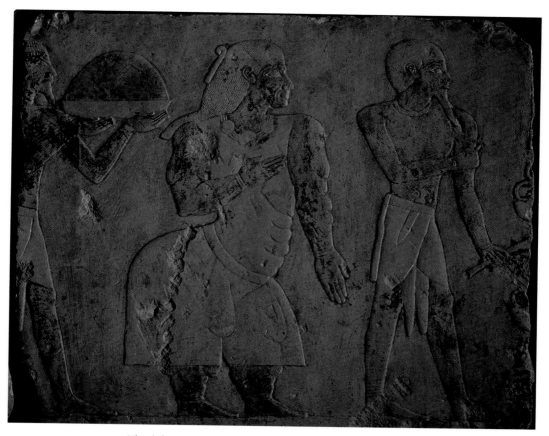

The deformities portrayed in this image of the queen of Punt, from the temple of Hatshepsut at Deir el-Bahri (18th Dynasty), have given rise to a number of explanations. The most plausible is that the queen suffered from the obesity and muscular weakness typical of Dercum's disease. But other possible conditions include hypothyroidism with myxedema, achondroplasia, and elephantiasis (lymphatic filariasis). Elephantiasis, a parasitic disease that still affects 120 million people around the world, causes the skin to thicken and fluid to collect in the extremities, producing the "elephant skin" visible here. Egyptian Museum, Cairo.

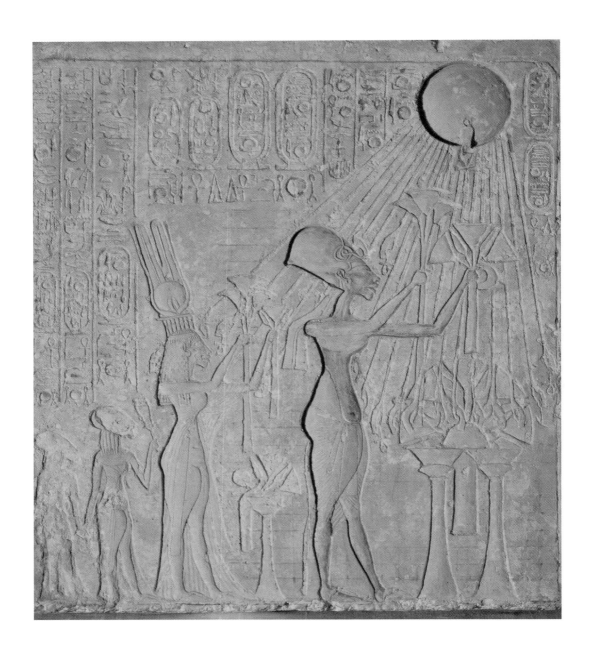

to argue that he was probably sterile, thereby casting doubt upon the paternity of the six daughters he is said to have had with Nefertiti. If he had any sons, as a legend maintains, none of them was formally recognized, and, unlike his father, Amenhotep III, Akhenaten did not keep a harem. Nor did he marry a foreign princess, already in his time a widely favored diplomatic expedient. Tellingly, perhaps, at an age when he could still have hoped to produce a male heir, he named his brother coregent—or so it would appear.[28]

The noticeably protruding chin and large ears in portraits of Akhenaten may be signs of acromegalia, while the eunuchlike appearance of these images, marked by testicular atrophy and gynecomastia, could point to Klinefelter's syndrome.[29] Other etiologies have been proposed as well, including testicular and adrenal tumors, and a paraneoplastic syndrome with LH-like secretion.[30] The depiction of a bearded Akhenaten on one ostracon challenges such diagnoses, however, and the prospect of one day being able to decide which one is accurate is further reduced by the absence of the pharaoh's mummy, whose discovery is unlikely. On balance the available evidence suggests that Akhenaten suffered from a complex endocrine disorder, the exact nature of which may be impossible to determine with confidence. It is in any case futile to speculate solely on the basis of artistic renderings that combine realism and symbolism in differing proportions.

When all is said and done, the key to the enigma of Akhenaten is probably to be found in physical examination of members of his family, particularly the individual buried in KV55 (possibly Smenkhkara) and Tutankhamun, who may be his brothers or, since the identity of the mother remains uncertain, half-brothers. Smenkhkara died at an early age (about twenty-five years) and without issue. His mummy, despite being badly damaged, reveals protrusive jaws and a somewhat gynecoid skeleton that agrees with pictorial evidence of a rounded abdomen and

The pharaoh Akhenaten making an offering to the sun god Aten. A variety of diagnoses have been proposed to account for Akhenaten's elongated fingers, protruding belly, and androgynous features: Klinefelter's syndrome, testicular and adrenal tumors, paraneoplastic syndrome with LH-like secretion, Marfan's syndrome. A more skeptical view is that the figure depicted in such images is not Akhenaten at all, but his queen Nefertiti, who may have acted as his co-regent. Painted limestone stele from el-Amarna.

hips and mild gynecomastia. The mummy of Tutankhamun, who also died young (about nineteen) and without issue, has a diameter at the level of the shoulders roughly equal to the diameter at the level of the hips. Here again the mummy confirms artistic representations showing very slight gynecomastia. Taken together, these mild anomalies in Akhenaten's probable brothers suggest the existence of a family disease. Nonetheless it must be kept in mind that in the artistic style of the period Akhenaten's physique was probably idealized. Thus Tutankhamun's successor, Ay, though he was not related to the pharaohs who preceded him, is shown on reliefs as also having a bulging abdomen and slightly enlarged breasts.

Some Neurological Anomalies

Our knowledge of nervous disabilities and malformations in ancient Egyptians, obtained mainly from the study of mummies, is fragmentary as well. The supposed hydrocephalus of certain subjects has given rise to considerable debate. D. E. Derry described a mummy of a young adult of the Roman Period whose cranial volume was roughly twice the normal size. It is probable that the young man suffered from hemiplegia (paralysis) on his left side, as the bones of the limbs and pelvis, more slender on the left than on the right, suggest.[31]

In other cases this diagnosis carries plausibility even though it has not been definitively established. As we have seen, the mummy of Akhenaten's successor, Smenkhkara—or rather what some believe to be his skeleton, found in a tomb furnished with objects bearing the name of Akhenaten's mother, Tiye—is modestly gynecoid, with a broad and slightly eunuchoid pelvis having a breadth of 11 centimeters at its highest point. Examination of the skull disclosed projecting jaws and large temporal bones, brows, and cheekbones. To account for these various symptoms Smith and Dawson proposed hydrocephalus without being able, radiologically or otherwise, to confirm their diagnosis.[32]

With regard to other malformations, one may cite the discovery, by Don Brothwell and A. T. Sandison, of a small anencephalic body in the midst of the mummified monkeys at Hermopolis, as well as several cases of spina bifida found by P. H. Gray in his radiological study of mummies. Two skulls, found at different sites in 1949, both exhibit hyperostosis (abnormal thickening) of the dome of the skull. One of them, dating from the 1st Dynasty, displays signs of an underlying tu-

Blindness is particularly well attested in representations of harpists, who were also apt to become hunchbacked as a result of their work. This blind harpist appears in a detail of a wallpainting in the tomb of Nakht, scribe and priest under Thutmose IV, in the cemetery of Sheikh Abd al-Qurnah in Thebes.

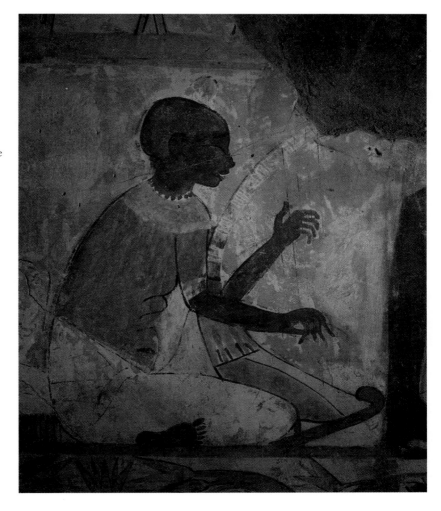

mor of the membrane enclosing the brain (meningioma); the other, dating from the 20th Dynasty, appears to present evidence of a tumor composed of lymph and blood vessels (angioma).[33]

Blindness

The theme of the blind musician, frequently encountered in Egyptian iconography, had a corresponding basis in medical knowledge. Several passages in the Ebers papyrus contain remedies for blindness *(shepet)*—but without indicating the cause of the particular condition requiring treatment (356–358, 420). Distinguishing between congenital blindness and loss of sight due to injury is therefore difficult. Elsewhere in the same papyrus reference is made to a related condition called *sharu* and its treatment by the application of liver, known today to be rich in vitamin A: "Another [remedy] for [the substances that cause] *sharu* in the eyes: liver of ox, roasted and pressed. Apply to [the eye]. Truly effective" (351). Or again: "Another [remedy]: liver of ox, placed on a fire of straw, emmer, and barley, smoked with their smoke. Press the juice into the eyes" (London 35).[34]

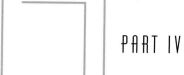

PART IV

PROFESSIONAL RISKS

8 Fishermen and Farmers

In order to form some idea of the many hazards to health in ancient Egypt, let us take a closer look at the sorts of conditions that physicians encountered in their daily practice. Inevitably doctors had occasion to question patients about the nature of their work, not only because the workplace constituted their principal environment but also because different occupations exposed workers to different risks. Taken together, these occupations tell us a great deal about the practice of internal medicine and surgery in pharaonic times.[1]

Fishing on the Banks of the Nile

With the exception of kings and priests, for whom the eating of fish was considered taboo, the Egyptians prized fish and caught them in great numbers in the shallow waters of the Nile and the marshes of the delta, where they waded through thickets of sedge and lotus, as well as in deeper waters off the coast, which they navigated on papyrus rafts.[2]

Under the Old Kingdom large-scale fisheries were established by the state and nets came to be substituted for harpoons and hooks made from bone and shell. Whereas the day's catch had once been carried directly, on poles or in baskets, to a chief of agricultural workers for inspection, now it was dried and packaged beforehand. But these advances hardly altered the conditions of life for fishermen, which remained very harsh. "These were ordinary people," Guillemette Andreu points out, "who worked in teams and were paid in kind a fraction of the total catch. Nothing set the fisherman apart from his fellows.

Like the oxherd, he came naked, carrying his rolled loincloth over his shoulders."[3]

Crocodile Hunting

The waters of the Nile were teeming with crocodiles. These animals terrified fishermen, who wore amulets for protection, and rendered their trade particularly dangerous. The *Satire of the Trades,* a popular work composed during the Middle Kingdom with the purpose of demonstrating the noble character of the scribal profession by comparison with other occupations, claims that "the fisherman . . . is more unhappy than [anyone] in any other profession [for] the place where he works is the river, among the crocodiles."[4]

The only real hope of security lay in capturing these ferocious beasts. Attempts were regularly made, as we know from Herodotus:

> Of the numerous different ways of catching crocodiles I will describe the one which seems to me the most worthy to report. They bait a hook with a chine of pork and let it float out to midstream, and at the same time, standing on the bank, take a live pig and beat it. The crocodile, hearing its squeals, makes a rush toward it, encounters the bait, gulps it down, and is hauled out of the water.[5]

Crocodile hunting was undoubtedly fraught with peril. From the Ebers papyrus we learn that the victim of an attack was treated with the following remedy: "What is to be done for the bite of a crocodile. If you examine the bite of a crocodile and you find it with the flesh mangled [literally, "pushed back"], while [the] two sides [of the wound] are separated, then you should first bandage it with fresh meat, as for every wound" (436).[6]

In addition to applying medicinal preparations, both the physician and the victim addressed prayers to the crocodile god Sobek.

Urinary Infections

Urinary schistosomiasis, a parasitical infection caused by the *Schistosoma haematobium* and transmitted by feces-contaminated water or by snails, is still endemic in Egypt today, affecting about 12 percent of the population.[7] In pharaonic times fishermen must have been the principal victims of this disease. The rarity of the condition in mummies suggests that people who could afford embalming, typically members of the upper classes, were largely untouched by it. But painted reliefs in

Bedwetting and First Teeth

of the body as the lesion in a manner consistent with Brown-Séquard syndrome.[36]

The same case in the Edwin Smith papyrus describes a locking condition ("the man whose head cannot be pulled away from the extremity of his shoulder") with neurological repercussions, notably spontaneous pain caused by attempts at cervical movement. It also mentions a series of craniocerebral wounds and fractures extending from the brain down into the sinuses that sometimes produce post-traumatic meningeal hemorrhage, and notes the danger of rhinorrhea or otorrhea associated with this type of fracture ("The man who loses blood from both his nostrils [and] both his ears, while he suffers from stiffness in his neck").[37]

A related case (Edwin Smith 31) involving dislocation of the upper spine ("the separation of one vertebra of his neck from another") leaves no doubt that Egyptian physicians had managed to discern the first two stages in the clinical picture of quadriplegia. In the first phase the patient presents a flaccid paralysis characterized by loss of feeling in all modes below the level of the lesion ("he is no longer aware of his arms and his legs"). This is succeeded by a second phase in which the paralysis becomes spasmodic and can cause urinary incontinence ("urine drips from his member without his knowing it").

Practitioners of the pharaonic period considered traumatisms of the skull and the neck to justify withholding treatment from patients, who were immobilized between brick or earthen supports and put on a light diet. Treatment was limited to the alleviation of symptoms, consisting of oil massages supposed to counteract contraction of the neck. It is more likely, however, that these massages helped to bring on death by causing subdural or extradural hematomas. In the meantime the neurological consequences of such injuries would have been horrible to endure.[38]

Remarkably enough, none of the medical papyri mentions trephination, the cutting out of disk-shaped parts of the cranium. Yet many skulls from ancient Egypt reveal lesions that seem to have been caused by surgical incision. The frontal bone of the skull of a princess of the 25th Dynasty, Horsiest-Mertamen, exhibits a circular perforation with beveled and perfectly healed edges—evidence that she underwent cranial surgery before she died. Two other trepanned skulls have been described by Ahmed Batrawi. Three more, from the Ptolemaic period, have been examined, as well as the skull of a mummy from the 18th Dynasty that, with the benefit of modern scanning techniques, discloses an oval deformation whose rounded edges likewise indicate that the patient survived surgery. These observations raise a number of questions, particularly with regard to the mode of anesthesia and the nature of postoperative care.[39]

Facial Trauma   During combat soldiers often received heavy blows to the front of the head. Fractures of the face are mentioned in several places in the medical papyri. An interesting case in the Edwin Smith papyrus concerning a complete or partial dislocation *(wenekh)* of the jaw describes a maneuver for reducing a dislocation of the mandible, or lower jaw.[40] Not only is the patient's inability to shut his mouth perfectly described ("his mouth [is] incapable of being closed"), but the technique of reduction is identical to the one that is still recommended today: "You shall place your thumb[s] on the extremities of the two claws [rami] of the mandible, inside the mouth, and your other fingers under his chin. You cause [the rami] to move downward so that they are put back in place" (25). Elsewhere in the same papyrus a fracture of the cheekbone is described with the same precision, as is a fracture of the mandible, recognizable by its crepitation: "This fracture crackles under your fingers" (17, 24).

Injuries to the ear, an organ of crucial importance in Egyptian physiology, were particularly frequent in combat. Edwin Smith 23 mentions the treatment of a wound to the ear sustained in battle, and several methods for treating such injuries are found in Ebers 766. The Egyptians believed that the breath of life entered the body through the right ear and the breath of death through the left ear, the former having been sent by the gods to provide the energy needed for the autonomous activity of the body, allowing the heart and the lungs to function independently of the will (Berlin 163g, 163h). This mythological context makes it clear why amputation of the ear was considered one of the most severe punishments.

The nose, for its part, was thought to permit the breath to travel down into the lungs and the heart, and from there to spread throughout the body via the vessels *(metu)*. The air that entered through the nostrils supported speech, thought, the will, and the dynamic currents that traveled through these vessels. As a point of entry for vital respiration,

A scene from the 11th–12th Dynasty tomb of two sisters, Senet and Khety, shows them standing beside a table covered with funerary gifts and inhaling the scent of lotus flowers, identified with the breath of life. The blue lotus (*Nymphaea nouchali* var. *caerulea*) was sacred to the Egyptians and figured prominently in ritual and in their pharmacopoeia. Amputation of the right ear, through which the breath of life was believed to enter the body at birth, was a punishment rivaled only by amputation of the nose, an organ that served as a conduit for vital spirits in later life.

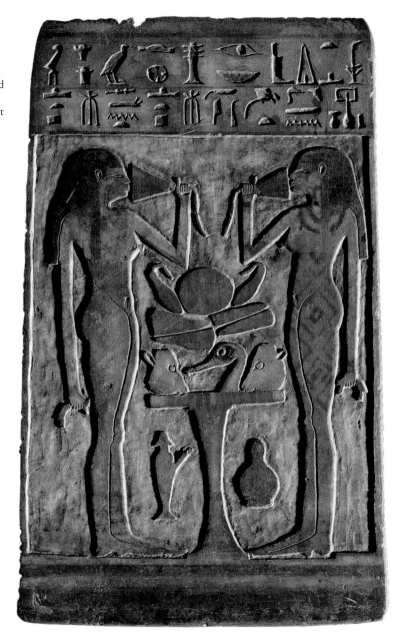

the nose figures in the opening chapters of the Bible: "The Lord God formed man of dust from the ground, and breathed into his nostrils the breath of life; and man became a living being" (Genesis 2:7). Among the Egyptians amputation of the nose was a comparably severe punishment to that of the ear, one that was inflicted on female adulterers in particular.[41]

Egyptian physicians may therefore have felt a special obligation to treat injuries to the nose, which were surely common during military training and combat. The Edwin Smith papyrus discusses fractures of the cartilage of the nasal septum and of its related bones, thus establishing a clear distinction between damage to the septum and damage to the bones themselves. In the first case a classic set of symptoms—edema, deformation, and bleeding—may be recognized:

> If you examine a man suffering from a break in the column of the nose, while his nose is crushed, while his face is indented, while there is a swelling on [the break] that protrudes, and while he has lost blood from both his nostrils, you shall say concerning him: "A man suffering from a break in the column of the nose. An ailment that I will treat." (11)

The proper therapeutic response consisted in plugging the nostrils with swabs of linen and then straightening the septum before immobilizing it—roughly the same treatment that is administered today:

> You shall clean [inside his two nostrils] with two swabs of linen [and then] place two plugs of linen, saturated with grease, inside his two nostrils. You shall then moor him at his mooring post until the swelling has gone down, and you shall [then] place two splints, covered with linen, thanks to which his nose will be compressed. You shall treat [the break] with grease and honey and vegetable tissue every day, until he is well. (11)[42]

In the case of a fracture of the bones of the nose, the following instructions are given:

> If you examine a man having a break in the chamber of his nose, and you notice that the nose is crooked, while the face is flattened [and] over [the break] is a swelling that protrudes, you shall say

Dead and dying soldiers at the Battle of Qadesh. This relief from the mortuary temple of Rameses II at Thebes captures the lethal fury of chariot assaults against massed ranks of infantry. The Edwin Smith papyrus gives the first known set of instructions for the diagnosis and surgical treatment of injuries to the head and upper body commonly encountered in ancient warfare.

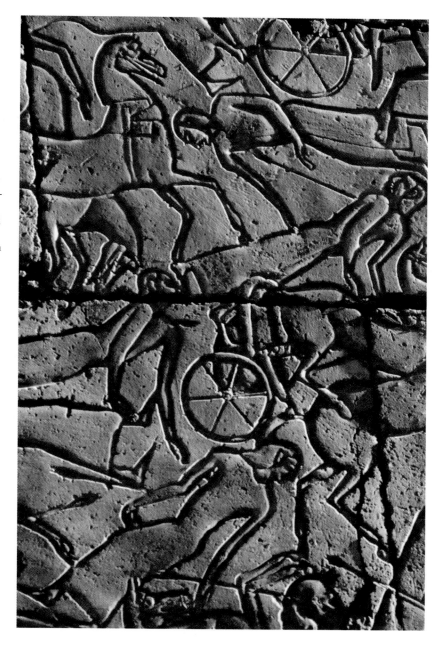

concerning him: "A man suffering from a break in the chamber of his nose. An ailment that I will treat."

... Next you shall put two plugs of linen saturated with grease in his two nostrils. [Then] you shall put two splints covered with linen. Bandage with that. You shall treat [the break] next with grease, honey, and vegetable tissue every day, until he is well. (12)

Mention is also made of an osseous rupture in the nose accompanied by a bloody discharge, probably as a consequence of a fracture of the otic bone. In this case, however, the physician concludes pessimistically: "A man suffering from an [osseous] rupture in the nose, an ailment that cannot be treated" (13).

The following case in the Edwin Smith papyrus directs the physician to suture a wound to the nostril ("You shall maintain together [the lips of] the wound with thread"), having first removed the coagulated blood ("You shall clean out every worm of blood that has clotted inside his nostril"), and then to apply a curative dressing of fresh meat (14).

Surgery in Wartime Small wooden and ivory labels discovered in the royal tombs at Abydos excavated by Sir Flinders Petrie in 1899–1901 may provide evidence of surgical intervention for nontherapeutic purposes. These labels were sometimes decorated with depictions of the jubilee festival *(heb-sed)*, at which the pharaoh was required to undergo certain trials to demonstrate his fitness to continue to govern the country after a reign of thirty years. In one scene it is possible to make out a seated figure holding a sharp instrument that is pointed at the throat or breast of another figure, who is kneeling with his arms behind his back. Between the two human figures is a vase. Some Egyptologists have interpreted this scene as a ritual sacrifice of a prisoner of war. Vladimir Vikentieff, however, argued that it illustrates a tracheotomy in which new life is symbolically breathed into the prisoner, who stands here for the pharaoh himself.[43]

Amputation, however, seems never to have been performed for therapeutic purposes. Instead, as Diodorus reports, it was a classic punishment handed down by a tribunal: "In the case of those who had disclosed military secrets to the enemy the law prescribed that their tongues should be cut out, while in the case of counterfeiters or falsifiers of measures and weights or imitators of seals [. . .] it ordered that both their hands should be cut off." In the course of the conspiracy trial involving members of Rameses III's harem, to give another example, two judges who had allowed themselves to be bribed were sentenced to amputation of the nose and ears.[44]

The same penalty was applied to enemies in war. Reliefs in the mortuary temple of Rameses III at Medinet Habu contain scenes in which the severed hands and phalluses of enemies killed in combat are counted in front of the king. Researchers have found signs of amputation in mummies as well. Don Brothwell and Vilhelm Møller-Christensen analyzed a forearm whose two bones were cut off above the wrist and rejoined by a large osseous callus. P. H. Gray examined a mummy whose forearm had likewise been severed above the wrist, to which a crude prosthesis made out of linen bandages had been attached after death by the embalmers.[45]

Royal Valor

Military campaigns brought suffering and death not only to soldiers but to their leaders as well. The medical cases of two kings fallen on the field of battle illustrate and summarize the dangers faced by combatants.

Seqenenra Taa, a pharaoh of the 17th Dynasty nicknamed "the Brave" for his prowess as a warrior, was a handsome man—tall, slender, and powerfully built, with black curly hair and a small, elongated head—who died a violent death at about the age of thirty. Radiological examination of his mummy showed the cause of death to have been six wounds to the skull and the face.[46] To be precise: a frontal, transversal, open fracture of the skull, about ten centimeters long; an open fracture of the rim of the right eye socket and another of the right cheekbone, probably caused by a battle-axe; an open comminuted fracture of the bones of the nose, probably the result of a blow from a stick (or an axe handle); another such fracture of the left cheekbone; and, finally, an open fracture of the left mastoid process, with damage to the first vertebra of the neck, due to a pointed instrument (perhaps a spear or a javelin). These lesions were caused by two types of weapons, one pointed and the other either blunt or sharp-edged, known to have been in use during the period both in Egypt and among the Hyksos.[47]

Further inspection revealed no wounds on either the torso or the arms, which suggests that Seqenenra did not resist for very long. The foul odor of the mummy (due to an insufficient quantity of natron), the

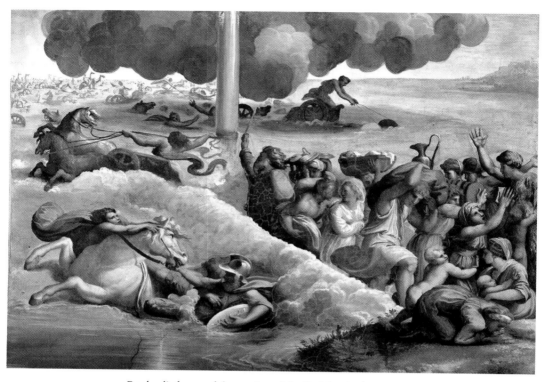

Raphael's fresco of the parting of the Red Sea, in the Vatican Palace in Rome, is perhaps the best-known illustration of the Hebrew Exodus from Egypt. Recent computer models confirm that changes in the force and direction of the prevailing winds could in fact have cleared a path for the fleeing Israelites and then suddenly caused a wall of water to fall back upon the pharaoh and his army.

fact that the brain was left in place, and the dislocation of limbs from overly tight bandaging all suggest that mummification was carried out in haste. This has given rise to two hypotheses. The first is that the king was assassinated in Thebes by members of his own entourage, dying from a dagger to the neck (possibly while he slept) followed by a succession of blows by club and axe testifying to the fury of his murderers. The second, more probable, explanation is that Seqenenra did indeed die a death worthy of his name on the field of battle, and that circumstances permitted only perfunctory embalming.[48]

Merenptah, though he is not named explicitly in either the Bible or the Koran, is thought by some authorities to have been the famous pharaoh of the Hebrew Exodus. In old age he was bald, toothless, and corpulent (if not actually obese), and suffered from cervical osteoarthritis and atherosclerosis. He died from the consequences of traumatic lesions. Yet for someone who is supposed to have been swallowed up by the Red Sea, his mummy seems strangely untouched by its waves. His corpse, like that of Seqenenra, displays an impressive record of injury: a craniocerebral wound; loss of cutaneous and osseous matter from the left metatarsus, the right clavicle, and the right first rib; a fracture of the surgical neck of the humerus; loss of bone matter from the tenth, eleventh, and twelfth right ribs; and comminuted fractures of both bones in the right forearm. This evidence suggests that Merenptah met his death in combat—but one wonders how an old man crippled by osteoarthritis could have chased the fleeing Israelites in his war chariot.[49]

Bakers, Priests, Scribes, Embalmers, Prostitutes

While the physically grueling labor required of farmers, fishermen, members of the building trades, and soldiers exposed them to the risk of particular injuries and diseases, more sedentary occupations carried health risks as well. Each profession presented physicians with a variety of conditions needing diagnosis and treatment, some of which were shared by the population as a whole. Here we take a brief look at five occupations that together tell us a great deal about the practice of internal medicine in ancient Egypt.

Bakers

The Greeks were quite right to call the Egyptians *artophagoi*—bread eaters—for bread and cereal products, mainly barley and wheat, made up the bulk of their diet. The corresponding importance of milling and baking in Egyptian society hardly needs to be emphasized.[1]

Dough was kneaded and formed into loaves—actually rather flat cakes, usually round but sometimes elongated—and placed in an oven constructed from three or four slabs of dried silt from the Nile, on top of which lay another wider slab. The dangerous nature of the baker's craft is described, no doubt with some exaggeration, in the *Satire of the Trades:* "When the baker is busy cooking and putting his loaves on the fire, his head is inside the oven, while his son holds him by the legs. If ever he slips from his son's grasp, he falls into the blazing fire." Apart from burns, the smoke pouring out of the oven exposed the baker to the risk of carbon monoxide poisoning. The likelihood that bakeries in ancient Egypt were very dusty as well would have favored the develop-

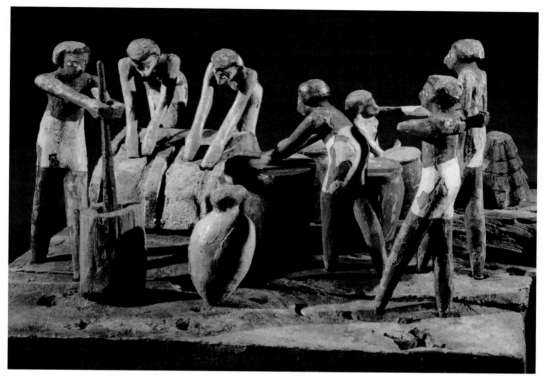

Wooden figurines from a Middle Kingdom tomb are shown grinding grain, kneading dough, and shaping and cooking round flat cakes of bread—which along with fish was the chief staple of the Egyptian diet. Analysis of loaves found in burial chambers has revealed the presence of stone particles and mineral elements, including sand, that almost surely account for the worn-down teeth found in mummies. Museo Egizio, Turin.

ment of asthmatic allergies to flour—an affliction still familiar among bakers today.[2]

Allergies and Burns   Bendix Ebbell was the first to propose that the medicinal recipes collected in a series of paragraphs in the Ebers papyrus (326–335) were meant to treat asthmatic attacks. In support of this view he cited the use in these texts of the word *gehu*, which includes a determinative that pictures a saurian—more precisely, a chameleon. Ebbell argued that the hissing sound emitted by this lizard in moments of danger connected *gehu* with asthma. The language in Ebers is too vague, however, and the treatments proposed too general, to justify so precise a translation.[3]

Notwithstanding the evident hyperbole of the *Satire of the Trades,* the danger of being burned from contact with the walls of the oven was quite real. The intense pain of such burns was bound to prompt recourse to magic. Some formulas were inspired by scenes from mythology, notably one in which the child Horus is treated for burns by his mother, Isis.[4] The milk of a woman who has borne a male child was often prescribed along with these litanies, again in allusion to Isis, the goddess who had nursed her son back to health with her own milk (Ebers 499–500, London 46). Another example of magical therapy called for third-degree burns (a "burned place when it decomposes"; Ebers 491) to be treated with a black plant tar whose color recalled that of the necrotic eschar, or scab of dead skin, that forms after this type of injury.

Some of the medical remedies employed are no less puzzling to the modern mind than the magical ones. Thus we read, for example, of a thick excrement-based paste applied as a dressing for first- and second-degree burns (Ebers 488, 498). What could be more surprising considering the risks of infection? The section on burns in the Ebers papyrus concludes with a recipe whose efficacy the author insists is attested by experience: "Truly effective! I have seen [it] and [it] has often happened for me" (Ebers 509). One infers that practitioners may well have placed a similar confidence in the medicinal use of excrement.

The damage to the skin caused by burns often remains visible after they have healed. One prescription addresses this problem from a cosmetic point of view, promising "to drive away white blotches due to the burned place" (Ebers 504).

Dental Attrition   Careful examination of mummies' teeth has revealed a general wearing down of dental surfaces, in persons of all periods and social classes, apparently caused by the Egyptians' extraordinary fondness for bread. Analysis of the composition of loaves that had been locked away with the deceased in their tombs yielded a wealth of information, and confirmed that the wearing away of the teeth was a consequence of chewing bread that contained substantial traces of abrasive minerals (sand, feldspar, mica, and sandstone).[5] This discovery may seem less surprising when one considers that minerals could have been inadvertently incorporated at each of the stages involved in breadmaking, from the harvesting of the wheat to the rising of the dough outdoors under the sun. In addition to minerals present in the earth in which it was grown, the wheat would have become mixed with flint from the sickles used in gathering it, with sand blown up by the wind during winnowing and storage, and with splinters of pestle or millstone during the crushing of the grain.[6]

Priests

Under the Old Kingdom, when the temples dedicated to the gods or to the funerary cult of the king had no permanent staff, priests did little more than perform occasional services and rites as the calendar required. The emergence of an established clergy at the end of this period coincided with the award of charters of immunity to the temples, partly or wholly exempting their agricultural estates from taxes and from corvée labor. Little by little an economy organized mainly around mortuary cults and worship of the gods grew up, and with it a professional class of priests. This class became progressively larger until finally, during the New Kingdom, it threatened to absorb the monarchy.[7] In addition to the staff of the temples (in which prophets made up the upper clergy, priests the lower), it included women as well as lay officials who were paid an hourly wage.[8]

"Upon entering the service of a particular divinity, in a particular temple," Philippe Martinez notes, "the priest took his place in a highly structured and diversified, often rigid hierarchy that was closed in upon itself and wholly autonomous, both with respect to the civil authorities and to other religious organizations." The sacred domains under the control of the clergy comprised not only the temple grounds themselves but also the great expanses of arable land that furnished food for worship and for feeding the temple staff. These dependencies constituted, moreover, both a form of transferable wealth and a source of income. The temple of Amun at Karnak, for example, the most important of them all, employed 81,322 men at the end of the reign of Rameses III.[9]

In many of these establishments one finds evidence of a corps of med-

This wallpainting from the 18th Dynasty tomb of Inherka in Deir el-Medina shows a priest holding two ducks as offerings. A sedentary way of life, combined with a largely meat-based diet from which fish was expressly excluded, may have exposed members of the priesthood to higher levels of cardiovascular risk than other segments of the population.

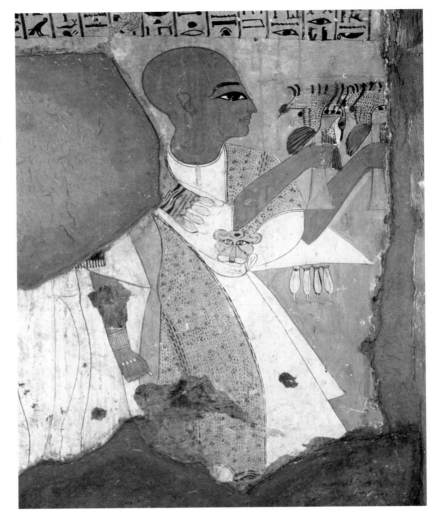

ical practitioners. Thus, for example, the Amherst papyrus describes a certain Pahatyu as "physician of the temple of Amun" in the seventeenth year of the reign of Rameses IX. Another doctor active during the 20th Dynasty, Innay, was overseer of physicians *(imy-r swnw)* at the temple of Ptah at Memphis. The name of Merye, chief physician *(wer swnw)* of the temple of Thoth and a native of Thebes, occurs in an inscription at Deir el-Bahri, and Padiamen, chief physician of the temple of Osiris, is mentioned on a stele from the Late Period. Herodotus tells us something about the way of life of their patients: "The priests shave their bodies all over every other day to guard against the presence of lice, or anything else equally unpleasant, while they are about their religious duties . . . they are free from all personal expense, having bread made for them out of the sacred grain, and a plentiful daily supply of goose-meat and beef, with wine in addition. Fish they are forbidden to touch."[10]

This account suggests that the standard of living of temple priests differed substantially from that of ordinary people with respect to hygiene and diet. The average daily ration of a worker during the Middle Kingdom, for example, consisted of two pitchers of beer and three loaves of bread.[11] At the same time, the combination of a diet that was rich in meat and poor in fish combined with a comparatively sedentary mode of life is likely to have produced higher rates of both tooth decay and atherosclerosis among the priestly class.

Cardiovascular Risk   A variety of representations and texts, even meals preserved in tombs, support the view that fish was a staple food for the poorest segment of the population, with meat (more often boiled than grilled) being reserved for feast days and other special occasions—especially beef, which was more prized than mutton, goat, or pork. Vegetables were part of the basic diet of Egyptians of all classes, who ate broad beans, chickpeas, and lentils in addition to radishes, cucumbers, pumpkins, gourds, melons (including watermelons); also garlic, onions, and leeks as well as fruits, among them grapes, dates, figs, and sycamore figs. Spices such as cumin, celery, and coriander were commonly used, but sugar was unknown. Wealthy families sweetened their diet with honey and occasionally with carob.[12]

Fish, however, was considered unfit for consumption by certain privileged castes, including priests. Not surprisingly, paleopathological examination of mummies has revealed evidence of atherosclerosis in members of the upper class. Obesity, a reliable indicator of risk for cardiovascular disease, is observed in portraits of a number of kings and royal attendants: Amenhotep III, Rameses III, Thutmose II, Merenptah, and Sobekemsaf II among pharaohs; the Old Kingdom high lector priest Kaaper, Prince Hemiunu (nephew of Khufu), and, during the New Kingdom, Neferhotep, the blind harpist of the Leiden Museum who is depicted in a seated position with three enormous rolls of fat. So overweight was the high priest and military general Masaharta at the time of his death, during the Third Intermediate Period, that his hands could not be crossed in front of his genitals in keeping with mortuary custom. In addition to various cases of atherosclerosis detected in the mummies of priests, one of the most famous examples of obesity is Rameses II, who nonetheless lived to be at least eighty, perhaps rather more.[13] In addition to his bulging, tortuous, and calcified superficial temporal arteries (which supply blood to the scalp), radiological examination has identified atherosclerotic calcifications of the femoral arteries and of the two internal carotid arteries.[14]

Nonetheless it is difficult to draw any firm conclusions about the broader incidence of atherosclerosis in pharaonic Egypt. Most of the mummies available to us for examination belonged in life to a privileged minority that can hardly be taken as representative of the population as a whole. Yet even if the exact extent of this pathology cannot be known, plainly diet cannot have been its only cause. Carbon monoxide poisoning, apparently common to judge from the traces of carbon found in the lung tissues of many mummies, must have figured prominently among the risk factors. Poor ventilation of smoke from heating and cooking in most homes no doubt contributed to the development of plaques in the arteries by depriving the tissues of necessary oxygen and thus increasing capillary permeability to lipidic substances.[15]

A more troubling and controversial question, over which much ink has been spilled, is whether nicotine poisoning was known in ancient Egypt. The discovery of tobacco in the abdomen of Rameses II during an exhibition in Paris in 1976 aroused widespread disbelief. If it was not debris left behind by a careless museum attendant, surely it must have been placed there by a mischievous scholar as a practical joke? But laboratory analysis later confirmed its authenticity. It is impossible to dispute either the botanical identification and dating of the substance found in the pharaoh's body or the presence in it of nicotine, along with the dermestes beetle, an insect pest specific to the plant genus *Nicotiana*.[16]

Patients suffering from atherosclerosis were treated with a variety of ointments intended to loosen, not the vessels themselves, but rather substances that were likely to harden inside them. One remedy in the Ebers papyrus recommended the following: "fat of bull: 1; wine dregs: 1; garlic: 1; charcoal from the walls [that is, soot]: 1; bryum [?] seeds: 1; pea seeds: 1; seeds of the *djas*-plant: 1; *sia*-mineral from the South: 1; terebinth resin: 1; incense: 1. Smear the outer flesh [with it] and put under the sun" (Ebers 657). The hardening, or rigidification, of the vessels was attributed either to normal wear or to an assault by harmful substances, hindering the free passage of corporal fluids, producing tension and painful pressure, and hampering movement. Contrary to the modern interpretation of atherosclerosis, while the Egyptians recognized that the vessels could deteriorate over time, it did not occur to them to consider whether their internal structure might be fundamentally altered in the process.[17]

Scribes

Without doubt the profession having the greatest prestige in ancient Egypt was that of the scribe, described by Guy Rachet as "the most privileged figure of Egyptian civilization."[18] In order to join the ranks of professional copyists and administrators, from the Early Dynastic Period onward, a child had first to learn the writing of signs in school.[19] After a long and difficult apprenticeship he entered the service of the pharaoh, in which scribes occupied an exceptional place: "See, there is no state in which one is not dominated, except that of the scribe who himself commands." The scribe was said to place himself "above all work and become a sage"; "his writing case and his roll [of papyrus] give him consideration and prosperity."[20] Exempted from taxes, excused from the forced labor that peasants and artisans owed the king, scribes were the indispensable agents of an unwieldy and complex system of administration, responsible for keeping accounts of cattle, harvests, and the output of craftsmen and workers. They were, in effect, the guarantors of Egyptian power and prosperity. And yet there is some reason to believe that they were not held in high esteem by the people, many of whom seem to have resented their privileges and above all their power to punish anyone who tried to steal property, or who could not pay taxes.

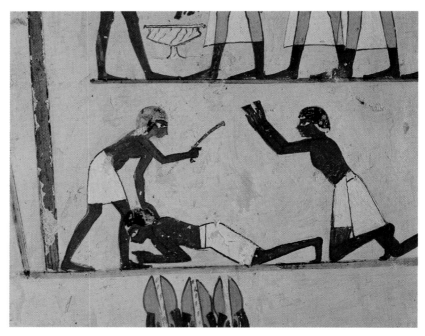

A slave being beaten by an overseer, from the 18th Dynasty tomb of Mennah, an estate inspector under Thutmose IV. Corporal punishment of freemen was often ordered by scribes, who were responsible for supervising the king's administrative affairs, monitoring payment of taxes, and imposing penalties for theft and malfeasance.

Dental Troubles It is hardly surprising that scribes should have suffered from poor dental health. They were paid in kind, in the form of bread, fish, and beer, a diet that was relatively poor in foods tending to inhibit tooth decay. Cavities, which were rather rare during the Predynastic Period, appear to have become more common in pharaonic times as a result of a diet that was much richer in cooked and sweet foods and that, beginning with the Old Kingdom, was consumed mainly by members of the aristocracy. Frugality, combined with the absence of foods that foster cavities, protected the poorer classes. Over time, however, the dietary habits of the upper class were adopted by the rest of the population, and tooth decay spread to all social groups. The incidence of cavities rose from about 3 percent of the population during the Predynastic Period to almost 7 percent toward the end of the Ramessid Period and perhaps as much as 20 percent during the Ptolemaic and Christian eras.[21]

The increase in tooth decay brought with it serious complications, as the study of mummies has once again revealed. Amenhotep III suffered from dental abscesses so disabling that the king of the Mitanni sought—without success—to intervene with the Syrian gods on the pharaoh's behalf. The mummy of Rameses II presents an enormous cavity in the first right lower molar, quite visible in X-rays, along with evidence of inflammation of the bone and detached fragments of dead bone (osteitis and sequestrum) from which he must have suffered horribly; indeed, this may have been the source of the blood poisoning from which he died. A skull from the 5th Dynasty displays an abscess of the second and third molars adjacent to the maxillary sinus. There is also mention of an "abscess (*benut*) in the teeth" in Ebers 746 (a condition translated by Lefebvre as "ulcer in the teeth").[22]

The premolar (or bicuspid) missing from the mummy of Sety I is one of a number of dental malpositions discovered in royal mummies. Ahmose-Nefertari, wife of Ahmose I, exhibits a protrusion of the upper jawbone, so that the incisors are projected forward, and an absence of wisdom teeth in the lower jaw—anomalies from which her grandmother Tetisheri seems to have suffered as well. The Papyrus Anastasi IV gives some idea of the suffering caused by dental problems, which the Egyptians could hardly have failed to take seriously. One worker was awarded a pension, paid out in wheat, in compensation for an ailment whose discomfort must have been obvious to anyone who looked at him: "All the muscles of the face dance, catarrh gets into his eyes, the worm gnaws at his teeth."[23]

It is unclear to what extent formal dental care was available in ancient Egypt. Dressings were made from several materials, in particular earth from Nubia, shaped to fill the decayed tooth. Temporary preparations of this sort, whose effectiveness depended on the characteristics of the materials used, were probably meant to suppress pain by sealing off the interior of the tooth from exposure to hot and cold.[24]

Dental extraction seems to have been widely performed—and by professional tooth-pullers, who have been identified in all pharaonic periods. A number of mummies display signs of healed bone with no lesion on either side of the missing tooth. The mummy of Merenptah, for example, has only six remaining teeth on the upper jaw and seven on the lower. The presence of a very regular mucous membrane above the bone suggests that the missing teeth fell out or were extracted during the pharaoh's lifetime. In some cases teeth were extracted from young people whose mummies otherwise display healthy dentition and well-healed bone.[25]

More surprisingly, archaeological evidence suggests that prostheses were sometimes used to hold teeth in place. The most interesting anatomical discovery, made in a tomb at Giza by Hans Junker in the 1930s, involves two teeth (the second and third left lower molars of a person who lived during the 5th Dynasty) that are tied together above their root by a braided gold thread 0.4 millimeters in diameter. Stained with tartar, they seem to have been implanted while the subject was still alive. But the wear to the two teeth, and the large space separating them, has cast doubt on the exact nature of the supposed prosthesis. Bernhard Weinberger argued it was a device intended to bring the wisdom tooth into normal occlusion. Others, however, incline to the view that the two teeth were bound together as an amulet.[26]

Other dental prostheses have been found as well. A bridge dating from the Ptolemaic Period was discovered in Tura el-Asmant. Another bridge, binding a canine tooth to a central incisor with the help of a gold thread, was discovered in 1952 in el-Qatta, northwest of Cairo, in an Old Kingdom *mastaba*-tomb. Radiography of a mummy in the Egyptian Museum in Cairo clearly shows a metallic thread that binds an unstable natural tooth to its neighbor in the upper jaw. But it is impossible to know whether this tooth was a true prosthesis or merely the work of an artistically minded embalmer, like the extremely fragile artificial teeth made out of ivory and mounted on wooden pivots found in certain mummies.

We also know of certain ailments of the tongue that cannot be precisely identified but that apparently were treated with mouthwashes and various medicinal preparations (Ebers 697–704). Like other offensive bodily odors, the bad breath that resulted from oral maladies disturbed the Egyptians, who were accustomed to suck on lozenges made from "incense, pine nut, terebinth, sweet sedge, cinnamomum, honey" (Ebers 853).

Mummies tell us little about pathologies of the stomach and pancreas, since for the most part they were emptied of these organs. We know more about the liver, an important organ for the Egyptians, which was carefully placed in a canopic jar during embalming. Even so, few hepatic diseases have been identified. Reliefs found in the tombs at Saqqara show figures with protruding navels, probably a sign of excess fluid in the abdominal cavity (ascites). A case of hepatic fibrosis of unknown origin was described by Marc Armand Ruffer.[27]

Diseases of the intestines, though very much in evidence in mummies, are known chiefly from the medical papyri.[28] The Berlin papyrus mentions abdominal discomfort ("his belly is heavy") in association with thirst ("he is thirsty during the night"), nausea ("he is covered with clouds like a man who has eaten the [unnotched *(nehet)*] fruit of sycamore"), and a blockage of fecal matter ("he is not regular in passing excrement")—all of which are signs of an intestinal occlusion ("[a] swamp formed by the wandering of burning substances") due to a fecal impaction ("his anus is heavy") (Berlin 154). It seems probable that both diet and sedentary habits would have favored the development of these conditions in scribes.

Paleopathological studies have shown that gallstones were exceedingly rare: only one case of biliary lithiasis (a priestess of Amun from the 21st Dynasty) was discovered among some 30,000 mummies examined by Elliot Smith and Warren R. Dawson; likewise a single case in 133 mummies subjected to radiographic analysis by P. H. Gray.[29] The rarity of this condition is very probably explained by the diet of the Egyptians, far less rich in fats than ours today, and by the relative absence of predisposing genetic factors. Scribes may have constituted an exception to this rule.

Two pharaohs warrant special mention here. The mummy of Rameses V presents an enormous inguinal hernia, and in Merenptah's mummy the scrotum is missing—no doubt having been removed prior to mummification, perhaps because of a strangulated hernia that had been operated upon with disfiguring results.

This painted lime-stone figure from the Old Kingdom depicts a scribe sitting cross-legged and writing on a papyrus. Freedom from manual labor and access to rich sweet foods make it likely that scribes and priests were more vulnerable than less privileged members of society to obesity, digestive troubles, and tooth decay. The Louvre, Paris.

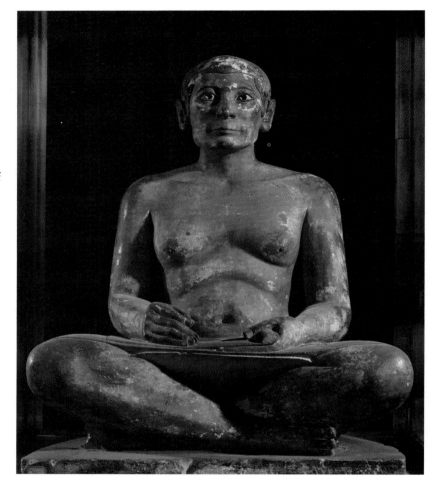

Constipation

We now arrive at the end of the digestive apparatus, and so of digestion itself. The Egyptians paid great attention to disorders of the anus, as we have seen, actually making it the focus of a medical specialty. Chester Beatty VI is devoted to anorectal disease, as are many paragraphs in the Ebers, Hearst, and Berlin papyri.[30]

It is reasonable to assume that scribes, at least as much as less privileged members of society, suffered from constipation. Recipes for combating constipation and "provoking defecation" were mainly composed of dietary fibers: broad bean *(gengenet)*, fruit of the *menuh*-plant, and *hiched*-fruit were all found to have a beneficial effect (Ebers 28, 36, 37). One also finds mention of a "dried notched fruit [*neqaut*] of sycamore"[31]—not the fruit of the sycamore tree we know today, it would appear, but of a variety of fig tree *(Ficus sycomorus)*.[32] Figs, which have a laxative effect when eaten raw, may have been used in dried form in herbal teas.

While constipation was surely common in ancient Egypt, as the abundance of recipes for its treatment suggests, the silence that surrounds diarrhea, whose frequency in Egypt is still well documented today, comes as a surprise. Mention is often made in the texts, however, of "cooling the anus" and driving out "burning substances [*kapu*] which are in the anus" (Chester Beatty VI, 18, 20, 22, 23, 24). It may be that anal fissures, or proctitis, resulting from diarrhea and dysentery are being referred to here. Elsewhere treatment with the aid of suppositories made of fatty substances is recommended: "Finely crush [this] into one thing, shape it in the form of a tampon and insert into the anus" (Chester Beatty VI, 6; Ebers 139, 140).

One also finds mention of a case of rectal prolapse (a "turning back of the anus") that was to be treated by a soothing remedy made from "flour of broad bean; salt from the north; goose fat; gum of barley" (Chester Beatty VI, 9.).[33] Rectal prolapses are frequently found in mummies, no doubt the result of abdominal expansion and distension caused by the gases produced during the body's decomposition.

Embalmers

We come now to the artisans of death, the workers of eternity. Embalmers included both *paraschistai* or cutters, who cut open the side of the body for evisceration using an "Ethiopian stone," and *taricheutai*, who were responsible for the body's actual embalming. Their workshops—known variously by names such as "house of perfection" *(per nefer)*, "place of purity" *(wbt)*, and "tent of purification" *(ibu)*—were located adjacent to temples and away from towns and cities, either for reasons of hygiene or from fear of the dead, whose place was on the western bank of the Nile, where the sun set. An ambiguous passage from Diodorus has been interpreted as evidence of a religious ritual or else of popular abhorrence:[34]

> Then the man called the slitter cuts the flesh, as the law commands, with an Ethiopian stone, and at once takes to flight on the run, while those present set out after him, pelting him with stones, heaping curses on him, and trying, as it were, to turn the profanation on his head; for in their eyes everyone is an object of general hatred who applies violence to the body of a man of the same tribe or wounds him or, in general, does him any harm.[35]

Nowhere else is mention made of such behavior, though we do know of a decree protecting cutters during the Ptolemaic Period, proof perhaps that they were discriminated against in some way.

With regard to embalming, not everyone was treated equally: pharaohs received special attention in their own temples, while lesser mortals were handled on an assembly-line basis, especially once mummification became available to large segments of the population. Nor was the conduct of the embalmers always free of scandal, if we are to trust the word of Herodotus, who mentions a case of necrophilia:

> When the wife of a distinguished man dies, or any woman who happens to be beautiful or well known, her body is not given to the embalmers immediately, but only after a lapse of three or four days. This is a precautionary measure to prevent the embalmers from violating the corpse, a thing that is said actually to have happened in the case of a woman who had just died. The culprit was given away by one of his fellow workmen.[36]

Inevitably embalmers were exposed to health risks in their professional tasks, no doubt similar to the ones that morticians face today. In addition to pathologies of the spine, arising from the need to lift corpses in restricted spaces and to carry them up and down stairs, workers were vulnerable to infection from contact with cadaveric fluids, which are rife with bacteria such as clostridia, as well as to irritative dermatitis from contact with the chemicals used in embalming. The smallest break in the skin allows entry to infectious agents that then go on to invade the digestive tract, lungs, and eyes. Moreover, as Daniel Moutet notes,

"The handling of a putrefied cadaver is extremely disagreeable. The gases of putrefaction, consisting of ammonia, mercaptan, and hydrogen sulfide among other compounds, have a very strong, revolting odor that quickly permeates clothing. There is no effective protection against it, and masks are totally useless." In ancient Egypt the moment of burial must have involved considerable psychological stress as well since some bodies were liable to break apart while being lowered into the grave.[37]

Cutaneous Infections Among skin ailments, embalmers are most likely to have suffered from boils, abscesses, and canker sores. Treatment no doubt proceeded along the lines indicated in a series of paragraphs in the Ebers papyrus (857–877), grouped by Thierry Bardinet under the title "Book of Tumors."[38] In the absence of specific details about surgical methods, we must be content with the recurring phrase "You shall operate upon it," or "You shall treat it as the *sa hemem* does," which suggests that Egyptian practitioners knew how to lance abscesses and hematomas using a bistoury or scalpel, and that they used cauterization to stop bleeding—perhaps even simultaneously making an incision to drain the accumulated pus or fluid and stanching the flow of blood with a heated lancet. A classic dressing meant to hasten the healing of the wound was then applied.

The Edwin Smith papyrus is more informative regarding the diagnosis, prognosis, and treatment of various infections of the skin. Thus, for example, it mentions a "head of abscess broken in his chest," marked by "swellings [that] have spread with pus over his breast, [and] have produced redness, while it is very hot when the hand touches it" (Edwin Smith 39, 46). Also an affliction that, according to Ghalioungui, may be an example of whitlow (or felon): "Remedy for a painful finger or for a toe . . ." (Ebers 616 bis).[39] This interpretation relies on the fact that, in Arabic, the word for whitlow *(dahes)* derives from the same root as the word for worm *(dohhas)*.

Parasitic Diseases Embalmers undoubtedly suffered from parasitic digestive infections, which we know were frequent in ancient Egypt. Traces of the worm responsible for strongyloidiasis *(Strongyloides stercoralis)* have been found in the intestines of the mummy Asru, dating from the 25th Dynasty, and, in another mummy, roundworm eggs associated with a case of ascariasis.[40]

The different worms mentioned in the medical papyri are difficult to identify in the absence of any generally accepted translation. Nonetheless it seems probable that the worms called *betju, hefat,* and *pened* correspond to ancylostomes (hookworms), ascarids (roundworms), and taeniids (tapeworms), respectively. None of these equivalences can be established with certainty, however.[41]

One recipe in the Ebers papyrus is accompanied by an incantation apparently intended to protect embalmers and their assistants from contamination:

> For the exorcism of *hefat*-worms: sedge *(isw):* 5 *ro;* pyrethrum: 1/4. Cook in honey and eat.
>
> Incantation: The *paut*-pieces [of the eviscerated mummy?] were separated and [the body] of the one who has lost his strength [the mummy] was returned. [Suddenly] a worm *(hery-shetef)* jumped in this the inside of my body. Whether it is a god who has acted, or a demon, may it be cast out! May the god undo what he has done in this the inside of my body. (Ebers 61)[42]

The Berlin papyrus contains a similar formula for keeping the same worm away from embalmers (Berlin 189). As a matter of rational medicine we know that pyrethrum, a member of the family Compositae of wild chrysanthemums whose roots possess anthelmintic and parasiticidal properties, would have protected them from intestinal worms found in mummies. The Ebers papyrus prescribes some thirty methods of treatment. Typical of this group is the following: "Another [remedy for the man who has the vermin]: root of pomegranate tree, crushed in beer: 5 *ro.* Let this rest in a *henu*-vase [450 ml] filled with 15 *ro* of water. You shall rise in the morning and strain this through a [linen] cloth. [It is] to be drunk by the man" (Ebers 63). The roots of the pomegranate tree are likewise endowed with antiparasitic properties, in particular against tapeworms and roundworms.[43]

Eye Disease

A final danger, and not a minor one, was posed by the splattering of chemical preparations during the embalming process, which would have reddened the eyes. What the Ebers papyrus refers to as "blood in the eyes"—whether due to hemorrhage, inflammation of the cornea (keratitis), or conjunctivitis—was treated in the following fashion: "Another remedy for driving out the blood that is in the eyes: two cups of clay, one with flour of *mimi*-wheat [*Triticum spelta*] and milk from a woman who has borne a male child, the other with [cow's] milk. Let [this] rest overnight beneath the dew. In the morning you [the patient] shall fill your eyes with this [spelt] flour. After that you shall wash your eyes with this milk, four times [a day]" (384).[44]

Prostitutes

Prostitution is often called the oldest profession in the world. Herodotus traced its origin to sexual relations between the gods and priestesses. The pharaoh Rhampsinitus, he relates, placed his daughter in a brothel to spy on its clientele.[45] Khufu (Cheops) is also said to have prostituted his daughter, in order to raise money for the construction of his tomb:

> But no crime was too great for Cheops: when he was short of money, he sent his daughter to a brothel with instructions to charge a certain sum—[my sources] did not say how much. This she actually did, adding to it a further transaction of her own; for with the intention of leaving something to be remembered by after her death, she asked each of her customers to give her a block of stone, and of these stones (the story goes) was built the middle pyramid of the three which stand in front of the great pyramid. It is one hundred and fifty feet square.[46]

Many prostitutes were also singers or dancers. One elderly scribe sought to warn his pupil against their charms: "Here you are spending all your time in the company of prostitutes, lolling about . . . Here you are next to a pretty girl bathed in perfume, a garland of flowers around her neck, drumming on your belly, unsteady, toppling over onto the ground, and all covered with filth."[47] The fact that these entertainers typically wore tattoos on the pelvis and the thighs has persuaded some scholars that they served the cult of the goddess Hathor.

Contraception

The risk of becoming pregnant was one that prostitutes sought desperately to avoid, all the more because abortion was punishable by death.[48] There is no doubt that women in ancient Egypt practiced contraception, for we know of at least six different methods. One recipe in the Ebers papyrus promised to make a "woman cease from conceiving for one

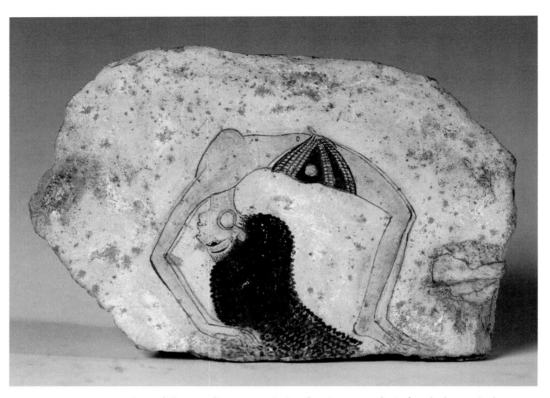

An 18th Dynasty limestone painting showing an acrobatic female dancer. Such entertainers often worked as prostitutes, possibly in the service of a divine cult. In addition to guarding against sexually transmitted diseases they had to take special care to avoid becoming pregnant because abortion was punishable by death. Museo Egizio, Turin.

year, two years, or three years: *qaa*-part of acacia; *djaret*-plant; dates. Finely crush [this] with one *henu*-vase of honey. Moisten a wad of vegetable fiber with it. Place [it] in her flesh" (Ebers 783). Other local methods of birth control, relying on a mixture of various ingredients with crocodile excrement (Kahun 21), may seem rather disgusting to modern sensibilities. One such preparation, smeared on a fibrous tampon and then inserted in the vagina (Ramesseum IV, C, 2–3), probably had a mechanical effect, obstructing the entrance of spermatozoa into the cervix. Several recipes called for honey, which would have served the same purpose by diminishing the motility of sperm. Another ingredient was acacia, whose fermentation produces an anhydrous lactic acid that, once dissolved in water, yields a compound known for its spermicidal action.[49]

Sexually Transmitted Diseases The phrase "vagina in which diseases develop" occurs in the Ebers papyrus (817)—probably evidence of vulvovaginitis, which is sometimes accompanied by discharges of blood and serous fluid ("like water at the bottom of which [there is the] like [of] cooked blood") (Ebers 831). This condition was treated by pouring a mixture of acacia, ox marrow, and several resinous substances into the vagina (Ebers 817). Other remedies are proposed to treat "burning substances that are in the uterus" (Ebers 820, 831), possibly the result of a genital infection. And the Kahun gynecological papyrus begins with a description of a probable gonococcal infection causing vaginal discharge and visual problems ("These are the uterine substances [called] . . . that are in her two eyes") (Kahun 1).

Elsewhere the mention of pains, and above all of the distinctive odor of burned flesh, has led some authors to conclude that the ailment described in the Ebers papyrus by the phrase "[woman] gnawed in her uterus, and in the vagina where [ulcers] develop" (Ebers 813, 814) may have been cancer of the uterus. Support for this hypothesis comes only from the genital malignancy discovered in a Ptolemaic mummy by A. B. Granville in 1825, an invasive tumor of the right ovary that had spread to the broad ligament of the uterus and the peritoneum.[50]

The Egyptians also appear to have been the first to describe prolapses and to treat them with resin-soaked tampons fitted to the dimensions of the vaginal cavity (Ebers 789). It is impossible to say with certainty whether or not the genital and rectal prolapses found in mummies were present before death.[51]

Menstrual Problems Menstrual disorders are repeatedly mentioned in the medical papyri. Amenorrhea, when it occurred in women who were not pregnant (the Ebers papyrus notes one woman "who has passed many years without her menstruation coming") caused much concern, and there existed at least three recipes for treating it (Ebers 828, 833; Edwin Smith verso 20).

A case of painful menstruation or dysmenorrhea, attributed in the gynecological section of Edwin Smith (verso 20) to an unidentified blockage ("bloody obstacle [in] her uterus"), is associated with abdominal pains and obstruction of the cervix by a pebble, polyp, or tumor. The discovery of an anomaly of the cervix suggests a true gynecological examination, but the treatments indicated furnish us with few details apart from the variety of ways in which remedies were administered, among them vaginal fumigation (Kahun 2, 20).

Epilogue:
Transmission of Egyptian Medical Knowledge

In combining an undeniable empiricism with religious and magical practices, the medicine of ancient Egypt may appear rather primitive from a modern perspective. Yet in its essentials it was not so very different from the tradition that prevailed in the Western world until the Renaissance. Little though Egyptian physicians may have known, as Gaston Maspero remarked, credit is perhaps due them for having known it thirty centuries before our era.[1]

Egyptian physicians were renowned throughout the ancient world. Homer described Egypt in the *Odyssey* as a fertile land where "the earth, the giver of grain, bears greatest store of drugs, many that are healing when mixed, and many that are baneful; there every man is a physician, wise above human kind; for they are of the race of Paeëon."[2] We know, too, that dignitaries from foreign lands came to consult the famed doctors of Egypt. In the Theban tomb of the scribe and royal physician Nebamun, who lived during the time of Amenhotep II, one finds a scene in which a Syrian prince presents Nebamun with gifts in recognition of his services. Herodotus tells us that Darius, king of Persia, brought the most famous Egyptian physicians to his court, and mentions the intrigues of an eye specialist sent by the pharaoh Ahmose II (Amasis) to treat Cyrus the Great, which persuaded Cyrus's son Cambyses to launch an invasion of Egypt:

> Cyrus had sent to Amasis to ask for the services of the best oculist in Egypt, and the one who was selected, in resentment at being torn from his wife and family and handed over to the Persians, suggested to

Cambyses by way of revenge that he should ask for Amasis's daughter in marriage, knowing that consent would cause the Egyptian king personal distress, and that refusal would embroil him with Cambyses.[3]

Herodotus also relates a famous instance, in which Darius was injured while dismounting from a horse, where the talents of Egyptian physicians seem to have failed:

> The injury was serious, the ankle being actually dislocated. It had been [the king's] custom for some time to keep in attendance certain Egyptian doctors, who had a reputation for the highest eminence in their profession, and these men he now consulted. But in their efforts to reduce the joint, they wrenched the foot so clumsily that they only made matters worse. For seven days and seven nights Darius was unable to sleep for pain, and was very ill.[4]

A physician from Croton named Democedes, who was a prisoner of the Persians—this at a time when, as Herodotus says, "the physicians of Croton were considered the best in Greece"—was then summoned to Darius's bedside. Democedes succeeded in healing the king "by using Greek methods and substituting milder remedies for the rough-and-ready treatment of the Egyptian doctors." Furious at having been maltreated by his court physicians, Darius sentenced them to be impaled. In the end they were saved by their Greek colleague, who pleaded with the sovereign to spare their lives.[5]

In Foreign Courts

A number of paleographic and archaeological sources tell of Egyptian physicians being sent to royal courts in foreign lands. From clay tablets discovered in the ruins at Tell el-Amarna we know that physicians were dispatched to several neighboring kingdoms, in particular the Near Eastern states of Mitanni and Ugarit. A message to Akhenaten asked that a doctor from his court be sent to treat a Mitannian prince named Shamsi Adad, who had no personal physician. Another text dating from Akhenaten's reign notes a similar request made by Niqmad, prince of the vassal state of Ugarit: "My lord, would that you send two Nubian pageboys and a physician of the palace. We have no physician here." In return, each of these rulers gave the pharaoh a statue of a local divinity renowned for its curative powers. Thus we have a letter to the aged and ailing Amenhotep III from the Mitannian king Tushratta, who sent the pharaoh a statue of the goddess Ishtar to hasten his recovery and to grant him long life. Gilles Boulu has argued that these countries did have their own native physicians, but none whose competence was comparable to that of their Egyptian counterparts.[6]

Other sources corroborate these records. Diplomatic correspondence between Egypt and the kingdom of Hatti a few years after the battle of Qadesh during the reign of Rameses II, found at Bogazkoy in central Anatolia, mentions the Hittites' urgent need for Egyptian medicine. The Hittite sovereign, Hattusili III, asked Rameses for a doctor to treat his sterile sister Matanazi. The pharaoh agreed, albeit with a certain skeptical reluctance: "Now see [here], as for Matanazi, my brother's sister, [I] the king your brother knows her. Fifty is she? Never! She's sixty for sure! . . . No one can produce medicine for her to have children. But, of course, if the Sun God [of Egypt] and the Storm God [of Hatti] should will it . . . But I will send a good magician and an able physician, and they can prepare some birth drugs for her [anyway]."[7]

A few years later a man named Kurunta, a vassal of Hattusili, also petitioned Rameses to send him a doctor. His request was granted: "Now I have summoned a learned physician. [The doctor] Pariamakhu will now be sent to prepare herbs for Kurunta, king of the land of Tarhuntas; he requested [a selection] from all the herbs, in accord with what you wrote to me." The Hittites' admiration for Egyptian expertise in herbal medicine is corroborated by a text noting that Rameses sent pharmaceutical preparations instead of physicians to Hattusili, who suffered from ophthalmia.[8]

Finally, there is the case of Rameses II's sister-in-law, the Bakhtani princess Bentresh, who according to legend suffered from a disease that the physicians of her country considered incurable. A delegation was sent to Thebes to petition the pharaoh to appoint a learned doctor capable of treating her. The royal scribe Djehutymes, who was probably also a physician, failed in this mission and announced that only the moon god Khonsu could save the princess. A statue of the god in his sacred bark was therefore sent to the king of Bakhtan, with the result that his daughter was healed. The sovereign considered keeping the divine effigy for himself until a dream persuaded him to return it. It should be emphasized that this account, though it may be loosely based on historical fact, needs to be regarded as literary rather than factual evidence.[9]

Diffusion of Medical Information

Foreign ignorance of pharaonic medicine was surely due in part to the Egyptians' strict secrecy about certain aspects of their sacred practices. Commercial activity had brought Egypt into contact with the ancient Near East since the Early Dynastic Period, however, particularly with the coastal cities of Syria and Palestine, and the presence of Egyptian physicians in foreign courts is likely to have encouraged the dissemination of medical knowledge.

Even if we lack direct evidence of encounters between Egyptian and Eastern physicians, it is reasonable to assume that the merchants who traveled the caravan routes between the Nile and the Indus Valley played an important role in the diffusion of medicinal plants. One gloss in the Ebers papyrus attributes a recipe to a foreign source: "Another remedy for the eyes revealed by an Asiatic from the city of Byblos" (422). The probability of such exchanges seems all the greater in view of the policy of conquest pursued by the pharaohs of the New Kingdom, as a result of which Egypt was able to extend its northern boundary as far as the banks of the Euphrates, on the outer edge of Mesopotamia. Among other things this would help explain the many similarities noted between Egyptian and Assyro-Babylonian medicine. The assumption of shared experience makes it natural, as Georges Contenau first pointed out, to interpret the obvious parallels between an Assyrian treatise on diseases of the stomach and certain paragraphs of the Ebers papyrus, for example, as evidence of a common approach to diagnosis and treatment.[10]

The Aegean World and the Greeks

By the end of the Old Kingdom commercial relations had been established between Egypt and Crete ("Keftiu"), and Egyptian physicians seem not to have been averse to borrowing from the botanical tradition of Cretan medical practitioners. Thus one recipe mentioned by the Ebers papyrus includes a "*gengenet*-bean (which is like the broad bean of the Keftiu country)" (28). There is evidence as well that Egyptian physicians used incantations in the Minoan language to exorcise certain diseases. The London papyrus, for example, speaks of "incantations for the Canaanite disease, what the [inhabitants of Keftiu] say in this case" (32). This disease was probably the lepromatous leprosy known in the Bible by the name of *sara'a* (Leviticus 13), a condition that was also rife in Syria, Palestine, and sporadically in the Egyptian delta. Hans Goedicke has suggested that Egyptian physicians may have employed the spell to protect themselves against this disease, which they noticed did not afflict the Cretans.[11]

Though Homer's testimony regarding the preeminence of Egyptian medicine had long been familiar to scholars, it was not until the beginning of the twentieth century that Egyptian contributions to Greek medicine were properly appreciated. Discovery of the "wall of the Milesians," a fortified trading post built in the eighth century B.C. in the Nile delta, furnished contemporary evidence of early commercial relations between the Hellenes and the Egyptians. Early in the 26th Dynasty, mercenaries from Ionia and Caria (today parts of Turkey) are said to have helped Psamtek I take power with the support of a fleet from the Ionian city of Miletus. According to Herodotus (2.154), the new Egyptian ruler expressed his gratitude to his allies by building a fortified settlement for them in the delta and leaving Egyptian children in their care to learn Greek and grow up to become interpreters. Contact between the two civilizations was deepened with the growing prominence of another foreign settlement, Naukratis, through which all Greek trade with Egypt was required to pass from 570 B.C., during the reign of Ahmose II. This city later became an important Hellenic cultural center and the site of both economic and intellectual exchange.[12]

Not only did Greece enjoy early and privileged contact with the land of the pharaohs, touring Egypt later became an obligatory pilgrimage for Greek scholars. Serge Sauneron has rightly emphasized the respect shown by the Greeks for Egyptian learning in spite of the persistent reluctance of the temple priests to disclose occult knowledge: "The ancient Greek texts leave no doubt that Egypt was seen as the cradle of all science and wisdom. The most celebrated Hellenic scholars and philosophers crossed the sea to seek initiation in new sciences by its priests. And [even] if they did not go there, their biographers hastened to include this voyage—now regarded as something both traditional and necessary—among the episodes of their lives."[13]

Among the earliest and most eminent of these scholars were Thales of Miletus (640–548 B.C.) and Pythagoras (580–490 B.C.), the latter being received by the pharaoh Ahmose II. Plato himself is said to have visited Heliopolis around 390 B.C., during the 29th Dynasty. Clement of Alexandria, writing in the third century A.D., put it nicely: "Plato went to Egypt . . . He who was all-powerful master at Athens . . . became a simple traveler and pupil."[14]

Representatives of the three principal schools of Greek medical thought, at Cos, Cnidus, and Croton, also established contact with Egyptian physicians. The resemblance between Cnidean and Egyptian ideas about the effects of disease on the body is particularly striking, and the "morbid principle" *(perittoma)* of the school of Cnidus, very like the Egyptian notion of *wekhedu*, may well be a case of direct influence.[15] Sais, the capital of the 26th Dynasty, was connected with Naukratis by a canal. It seems more than likely that Cnidean physicians living in Naukratis were able to communicate with their Egyptian counterparts at the famous medical school at Sais by means of interpreters. The itinerant Greek physicians and pedagogues known as *periodeutai* who traveled throughout the ancient Near East no doubt also came into contact with Egyptian practitioners. Awareness of Egyptian medicine would have spread to Croton, for example, with the story of Democedes' intercession on behalf of his Egyptian colleagues at the Persian court.

Hippocrates (460–377 B.C.), the celebrated leader of the school of Cos, was himself influenced by Egyptian medical thought. One rather doubtful legend relates that after being taught by his father and grandfather he traveled for three years in Egypt, going to the temples of Imhotep and Serapis at Memphis, where he absorbed the wisdom of the priests and scribes and perfected his skill not only in medicine but also in the art of interpreting dreams.[16] However this may be, the Hippocratic treatises certainly contain a number of borrowings from Egyptian medicine, including three methods for forecasting birth taken almost in their entirety from the Carlsberg papyrus, as well as a paragraph on the origin of sperm, which was said to be located in the spine.[17]

Hippocrates' somewhat confused description of the cardiovascular system may also have been inspired by the Book of the Heart in the Ebers papyrus. Moreover, the phrasing of certain Hippocratic maxims recalls the language of the medical papyri. In *On Joints*, for example, one finds the injunction to "study incurable cases so as to avoid doing harm by useless efforts," and in the *Aphorisms* the advice that "it is better to give no treatment in cases of hidden cancer"—echoes of the famous prognostic formula of the Edwin Smith papyrus, "an ailment for which nothing can be done."[18] Elsewhere, when Hippocrates recommends that a patient be left alone, one thinks of the memorable instruction in the same papyrus, "moor him at his mooring post."[19]

The exchange of medical knowledge seems to have continued in Ptolemaic Egypt, though probably with reduced intensity. Alexandria, founded by Alexander the Great in 331 B.C., rapidly became the cultural center of the Hellenistic world. In addition to the Museion and its celebrated library, created by Ptolemy I and containing perhaps as many as 700,000 papyri in the first century B.C., a famous medical school grew up there under the direction of Herophilus (who in defiance of Greek and Egyptian taboos performed the first dissections of human cadavers in the ancient world) and Erasistratus. Even though the Greeks generally showed little interest in local culture, and although, as Jean Yoyotte has pointed out, "the bulk of Egyptian information detectable in the Hippocratic corpus goes back, no doubt authentically, to borrowings prior to Alexander," the school of medicine in Alexandria was not cut off from all contact with Egyptian physicians.[20]

Greek borrowings from Egyptian medicine during the Ptolemaic Period were mainly of a technical character. Thus a Greek papyrus dating from the second century B.C. mentions a preceptor learning Egyptian in order to teach the language to young Greek slaves being trained in a school of medicine directed by an Egyptian specialist in the administration of enemas. This document is interesting, too, for its suggestion that Greek physicians were careful to avoid Hellenizing Egyptian medicine. Moreover, prescriptions on Greek medical ostraca found in Ptolemaic Egypt do not consist of translations from contemporary Egyptian sources, but rather repeat Hippocratic formulas—further evidence that Egyptian influence upon the development of Greek medicine occurred mainly in the pre-Hippocratic period.[21]

Hebraic Medicine

The prolonged stay of the Hebrews in Egypt during the late second millennium B.C. left its mark not only on their daily way of life and their vocabulary but also on their medicine.[22] There are many points of similarity between the five Mosaic books of the Pentateuch and the pharaonic medical papyri, particularly with regard to obstetric techniques, circumcision, and the prevention of epidemics. Thus, for example, Exodus 1:15–16 mentions Egyptian women giving birth in a squatting position with the feet placed on two bricks: "Then the king of Egypt said to the Hebrew midwives . . . 'when you serve as midwife to the Hebrew women, and see them upon the birthstool.'"

The Pentateuch is generally thought to have been written in the eighth and ninth centuries B.C., but its origins may in fact go back to the period of Hebrew captivity in Egypt. It is at least arguable that the Hebrews had a comprehensive knowledge of Egyptian medical practice, even if Egypt was not one of the principal sources—some scholars have claimed *the* principal source—of the books of wisdom of Israel.[23] Certainly remarkable coincidences can be observed in the domain of medicine, not least with regard to circumcision and mortuary customs. Thus it is said in the Bible that Zipporah, the wife of Moses, "cut off her son's foreskin" (Exodus 4:25).[24] Jacob himself was embalmed (Genesis 50:2–3), and the mourning lasted for seventy days, which is to say thirty days longer than the time required for the natron to dry out the body ("forty days were required for it, for so many are required for embalming").[25]

One notes, too, that a remedy for a disease of the eyes mentioned in one of the apocryphal books of the Bible, the Book of Tobit (6:4–12)—an ointment of bile—is strikingly like ones found in the Ebers papyrus (Ebers 347, 360). Similar names are given to certain ailments as well: the *sechepen*-disease of the skin[26] is called *schechin* in Hebrew, and the Egyptian word for vomiting, *qaa* (or *qas*) in the Kahun papyrus (192), recalls the biblical *qu'ah*. With the fall of the kingdom of Judah a number of Hebrew settlements were established along the Nile, for example at Elephantine in the sixth century B.C., but it is probable that the sizable Jewish community in Alexandria during the Ptolemaic Period, which included many physicians, played the leading role in the transmission of Egyptian medical knowledge.[27]

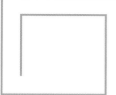

Primary Sources for Egyptian Medicine

The main historical sources are medical papyri, ostraca, epigraphic inscriptions and graffiti, and works of art, supplemented by the testimony of the travelers of Greco-Roman antiquity, biblical accounts, and the modern analysis of mummies. These materials are sometimes fragmented or otherwise incomplete owing to the extensive damage wrought by both nature and human beings over the past 5,000 years. The best-known example is the fire that destroyed the great library of Alexandria, which may have contained as many as 700,000 works in the time of the famous Cleopatra (Cleopatra VII Philopater).[1]

The Medical Papyri

The accounts of Greek travelers in Egypt, though their truthfulness has often been a matter of dispute, constituted the principal source of direct or indirect knowledge before the deciphering of the Egyptian language in the early nineteenth century. It was not until 1853 that Heinrich Brugsch made the first translation of a medical papyrus. Dominique Spaeth has described the problems involved in translating these documents, which are associated with the very structure of the Egyptian language and writing system, as well as the difficulty of determining the meaning of certain words, notably botanical terms.[2]

Egyptologists set about these challenging tasks using two methods. The first (and more reliable) of these exploited the connection between Coptic script and Egyptian hieroglyphics, as Jean-François Champollion had done to determine basic Egyptian vocabulary. The second method involved seeking common roots for words in Egyptian,

Greek (many Greek authors, notably Dioscorides, used the original Greek names for plants in their writings), Hebrew (which bore traces of the Jews' long stay in Egypt), and Arabic (which modified ancient Egyptian botanical terms only slightly).[3]

Though they are more often than not copies of older texts, the medical papyri provide the most authentic record of medical thought and practice in pharaonic Egypt. Nonetheless it is difficult to form a complete idea of Egyptian achievements on the basis of this collection of fragmentary texts—all the more since they are, as Thierry Bardinet has observed, "essentially practical manuals composed to allow a physician to diagnose pathologies in his daily practice and propose a suitable treatment. They are not theoretical treatises in the modern sense of the term—they do not explain illnesses—and, for this reason, a physician of the twentieth century is likely to find them inaccessible."[4]

The Ebers Papyrus   Conserved today in the library at the University of Leipzig, this is the longest and the most important of the medical papyri that have so far been discovered. It owes its name to the German scholar Georg Ebers (1837–1898), who bought it in 1872 from an Egyptian who claimed to have found it ten years earlier between the legs of a mummy in a tomb at Thebes. Three years later Ebers published a facsimile edition.[5] Translations followed, notably a German version by Walter Wreszinski in 1913 and an English version by Bendix Ebbell in 1937.

The papyrus is more than 20 meters long and 30 centimeters wide and consists of 108 pages of 20–22 lines each, numbered 1 to 110 (there is a gap of 2 pages after page 27, which is followed by page 30). The text, written in hieratic, dates from about 1500 B.C. during the reign of Amenhotep I. Nonetheless it almost certainly is a copy of an older treatise: grammatical constructions as well as a section containing remedies for hair loss, some of which have been found in a manuscript from the 6th Dynasty (about 2300 B.C.), point to an original date of composition during the Old Kingdom.

Its 875 paragraphs are juxtaposed without regard for logical order and constitute mainly a treatise on pharmacology and therapeutics, with a minor emphasis on clinical description (only 47 remedies include diagnoses). Some of its chapters, such as the Book of the Heart, are among the most important documents in the history of medicine. The historical interest of the papyrus is therefore considerable, not least for demonstrating that the spirit of rational medicine already existed long before the appearance of the first Greek physicians.[6]

The Edwin Smith Papyrus

Currently conserved at the New York Academy of Medicine, this papyrus was acquired in 1862 by a young American Egyptologist, Edwin Smith, from a merchant in Luxor named Mustafa Agha.[7] After Smith's death in 1906, his daughter gave the papyrus to the New York Historical Society. Responsibility for translating it was entrusted to James Henry Breasted, director of the Oriental Institute at the University of Chicago, who published a two-volume edition with commentary in 1930. Dating from the early 18th Dynasty, it may have come from the same tomb in the Theban necropolis as the Ebers papyrus. It is in any case very probably also a copy of an earlier papyrus: the grammatical structure of the text suggests a date near the beginning of the Old Kingdom.[8]

The papyrus consists of 12 pages, 4.68 meters in length and 33 centimeters wide, covered with hieratic script. Titles are written in red ink and the body of the text in black. In tone and approach it is more rational than the Ebers papyrus, including only one reference to magic (this in a case judged to be hopeless), and treats surgical pathology in a remarkably well organized and logical way. Beginning at the top of the head and moving downward (skull, face, neck, clavicles, shoulders, chest, spinal column), 48 cases describe traumatisms of the bones and soft tissues. Each observation unfolds according to a precise and fixed pattern: clinical description is followed by a diagnosis, then a prognosis, and finally the type of treatment to be administered.

The Hearst Papyrus

Discovered in 1899 during excavations at Deir el-Ballas, this papyrus was acquired two years later by the Hearst expedition to Egypt led by George A. Reisner, who published the hieratic text in 1905. A German translation was published by Wreszinski in 1912.[9] The papyrus is now the property of the University of California. Very probably written during the reign of Thutmose III in the 18th Dynasty, it contains 260 paragraphs with medical recipes for treating various afflictions of the skin, heart, bladder, and chest; dental ailments; parasitic diseases; the loss and whitening of the hair; bites; and fractured limbs. A number of these prescriptions are also found in the Ebers papyrus.

The Berlin Papyri   The work known as the Berlin papyrus (no. 3038), conserved at the Aegyptisches Museum in Berlin, consists of 204 paragraphs and dates from the 19th Dynasty. Discovered by Giuseppe Passalacqua in a terra-cotta vase buried ten feet under the desert sands near Saqqara, it was published in a German edition by Wreszinski in 1909. It is the only signed medical text that has survived, at least to judge from a note in one paragraph: "It was the scribe of sacred writings, the chief of excellent physicians, [who made] the book."[10]

Part of another medical papyrus, also in the museum's collection and sometimes referred to as the "small" Berlin papyrus (no. 3027), consists of some 15 pages written in 1450 B.C. or so, during the 18th Dynasty, that contain magical incantations for the protection of mothers and children as well as a treatise on infantile diseases. Ange Pierre Leca has described it as the "oldest pediatric treatise" known to us.[11]

A third, somewhat later papyrus held by the Aegyptisches Museum (no. 13602), written in demotic and dating from the first century B.C., contains prescriptions for preventing pregnancy.

The Kahun Papyrus   This papyrus, now conserved at University College of London, was discovered by Sir William Matthew Flinders Petrie in 1889 in very poor condition near the village of Lahun, in the Faiyum, among the ruins of the pharaonic residence at Kahun. Restored and translated by Francis Griffith in 1898, it is thought to be the oldest medical papyrus that has come down to us, having been composed during the reign of Amenemhat III of the 12th Dynasty (about 1850 B.C.). It is mainly a treatise on gynecology and obstetrics with a section concerning veterinary medicine (written in hieroglyphics).[12]

The London Medical Papyrus   Of unknown origin, this papyrus was acquired by the British Museum in 1860 from the Royal Institution of London and translated into German by Wreszinski in 1912. Dating from about 1350 B.C., during the reign of Tutankhamun, and measuring 1.25 meters in length and 17.5 centimeters wide, it is a collection of magical formulas containing 63 prescriptions for the treatment of diseases of the eyes, gynecological complaints, and especially burns.[13]

The Chester Beatty Papyrus VI	This papyrus from the 19th Dynasty, dating from about 1300 B.C. and no doubt copied from an older text, was part of a cache of documents found in excavations of Deir el-Medina that were eventually deposited in collections in England, Ireland, and Egypt. The recto is a treatise on diseases of the anus; the verso contains formulas concerning disorders of the breasts, heart, and bladder, as well as incantations. The papyrus is conserved in the British Museum.[14]
The Magical Papyri of Leiden	These two papyri (nos. I 343 and I 345), discovered at Thebes and now conserved at the University Museum of Leiden, date from the 18th and 19th Dynasties respectively. Both are copies of an older text and contain mainly remedies and magical formulas against various (and for the most part unspecified) conditions.[15]
	A separate text dating from the third century A.D., the Demotic Magical Papyrus of London and Leiden, was translated into English by Griffith and Thompson in 1904.[16]
The Brooklyn Papyrus	These two manuscripts (Brooklyn Museum 47.218.48 and 47.218.85), dating from the 30th Dynasty (about 350 B.C.), constitute a single papyrus that amounts to a veritable treatise on herpetology and ophiology. It describes various reptiles and the consequences of their bites and provides guidance for the treatment of victims.[17]
The Carlsberg Papyrus VIII	Of unknown origin, this document was published for the first time in 1939, in English, by Erik Iversen. Three fragments written in hieratic go back to the 19th and 20th Dynasties.[18] Currently conserved at the Egyptological Institute of the University of Copenhagen, it contains mainly gynecological prescriptions and material concerning pregnancy.
The Ramesseum Papyri III, IV, and V	These papyri, published by Alan Gardiner in 1955, were discovered in 1896 by James Quibell in a tomb of the Middle Kingdom near the Ramesseum. Papyrus III concerns ocular diseases and illnesses of children; IV, illnesses of women and children; and V, vascular disorders. They are of mixed medical and magical content (with the exception of

V, which is purely medical) and originally belonged to the private library of a learned man of the 12th Dynasty.[19]

Other Papyri A number of other papyri are either wholly or partly medical. These include the Amherst papyrus; the Cairo papyrus; the Anastasi papyrus; the Insinger papyrus, an important Late Period demotic wisdom text, which deals with the nature of God and human morality; the Louvre papyrus (E. 4864), a medical text written on the verso of the magico-religious papyrus no. 3279, also conserved at the Louvre, which concerns remedies for vascular disorders and *hefat*-worms; the Westcar papyrus, which deals with childbirth; the Vatican papyrus, containing anatomical lists for the protection of parts of the human body; and the Vienna papyrus (no. 6257), also known as the Crocodilopolis Medical Book, a demotic manuscript from the second century A.D. that contains a comprehensive pharmacopoeia.[20]

The so-called Turin Canon, a Ramessid document from the thirteenth century B.C. that is the most informative of the royal chronologies (or "king-lists") and the only one to have survived in papyrus form, was translated into English by Gardiner in 1959.[21]

Other Primary Sources

Medical Ostraca Ostraca contain succinct statements about the type of treatment prescribed for a given ailment as well as texts of incantations. Spaeth has inventoried the various items so far discovered:[22]

- Cairo 1091 is a limestone flake that contains three remedies: one for driving out suffering, another for cough, and a third concerning the heart.
- London 297, found at Tell el-Amarna, says simply to "smear the patient with the fat of a bull."
- Louvre 3255 is a piece of glass on which are inscribed medical formulas for the treatment of earaches.
- Berlin 5570 dates from the Roman Period and contains six medical formulas for ointments.

- The C. I. Milne ostracon contains an incantation for protection of the limbs based on the principle of similarity.
- Deir el-Medina 1091 is a prescription "for curing all illnesses."
- The Ramessid ostracon of Thebes bears an incantation against the demons responsible for a disease.
- Ramesseum ostracon 35 records a spell for use against snake bites.

Archives, Inscriptions, and Rock Carvings

Other sources of information include political archives, mural inscriptions, funerary stelae, and mortuary objects. Cuneiform tablets found at Tell el-Amarna recording the correspondence of Rameses II with Hittite sovereigns, for example, mention health problems in addition to the names of individual physicians. Inscriptions in the tombs not only of physicians, but also of high officials whom they treated, have made it possible to identify a great many doctors and to learn about their careers and the composition and structure of the medical profession in ancient Egypt. The tombs of Akhhotep and Irenakhty at Giza, and of Mereruka at Saqqara, are particularly revealing in this regard. Additionally, epigraphic evidence found in tombs at Saqqara and Deir el-Medina has cast valuable light on a variety of diseases and congenital deformations. Commemorative stelae (such as those of the first known physician, Hesyra, now in the Cairo Museum, and of the 19th Dynasty physician Iuny, in the Ashmolean at Oxford and the Louvre), sarcophagi (such as that of the 12th Dynasty physician Gua, in the British Museum), and statues (such as that of the 26th Dynasty physician Psamteksoneb, in the Vatican) have yielded further information. The famous funerary stele of the Syrian doorkeeper Roma, now in the Carlsberg Glyptotek Museum in Copenhagen, is reproduced elsewhere in this book.

A number of rock carvings of medical interest, mostly the work of members of expeditions to mines and quarries, mention the presence of physicians. The best-known figures are Heryshefnakht, whose titles and activities are described in a graffito found in the alabaster quarries of Hatnub, and his subordinate Ahanakht.[23]

Works of Art

Egyptian art—drawings, bas-reliefs, and statues representing persons suffering from medical conditions, surgical instruments, and so on— constitutes a valuable source of documentation for the historian of medicine. Tombs cut into desert cliffs during the Middle and New Kingdoms contain mural paintings of individual physicians.[24] The Roman Period temple of Kom Ombo is especially noteworthy for its depiction of some four dozen surgical instruments, many of which have been identified with a high degree of probability.[25] The discovery of medical, surgical, and pharmaceutical objects (including anthropomorphic containers and jars containing ointments) has improved our knowledge of Egyptian medicine as well.[26]

Interpreting the Ten Plagues of Egypt

A number of accounts, and in particular the one found in the Old Testament, have preserved the memory of ancient Egypt over the centuries. The adoption of the infant Moses, found in a basket on the banks of the Nile by the pharaoh's daughter, and the "ten plagues of Egypt" that led to the Hebrews' escape from captivity across the Red Sea are among the best known of all the stories of the Bible. This titanic struggle set Moses and his brother Aaron, fortified by their faith in the god of Israel, against the pharaoh himself, the earthly representative of the sun god Ra, and his magician-priests. Amplified, dramatized, and stylized in the biblical account, the story of the Exodus occupies a special place in the history of the Hebrews, symbolizing the clash between two peoples, two cultures, and two conceptions of divinity that ended in complete rupture.

Four centuries after Joseph and his brothers settled in the land of Goshen to the east of the Nile delta, a region renowned for its fertility, the tribes of Israel had given up a nomadic existence in favor of a settled life as herdsmen and farmers on lands granted them by the pharaoh in return for an annual tithe amounting to one-fifth of their produce (Genesis 41:34). In the course of their stay in the valley of the Nile the descendants of Jacob, who until then had lived in tribes and clans, became unified as a nation worshipping a single god, Yahweh. During the sixteenth century B.C., however, the situation of the Hebrews in the land of Goshen, peaceable up until then, suddenly and without warning deteriorated.

Alarmed by the Hebrews' high birth rate, which made him fear that they might ally themselves with Egypt's enemies, the pharaoh forced them to leave their pasture lands and enlisted their labor in building the kingdom's new capital, Piramesse. Furthermore, to limit the growth of the subject population, he ordered Egyptian midwives to drown all its newborn male children. It was in this atmosphere of hardship and persecution that Moses was born, about 1300 B.C., and cast adrift in the famous basket made of bulrushes on the edge of the Nile. Rescued by the pharaoh's daughter, Moses was raised in the royal palace, where he acquired a thorough knowledge both of Egyptian culture and of the mind of the pharaoh himself, who assigned a fundamental importance to dreams and omens.

It was only on attaining adulthood that Moses was informed of his origins and made aware of the sufferings of his people. After an altercation in which he killed an Egyptian foreman who had assaulted a Hebrew, Moses took refuge for forty years in the land of Midian, east of Akaba. Then the vision of the burning bush caused him to return to the land of Goshen to plead with the pharaoh to let his people leave Egypt. Unwilling to lose an important part of his labor force, the pharaoh refused. Moses responded by transforming his brother Aaron's rod into a serpent (Exodus 7:10–12) as a symbolic demonstration of the power of the god of Israel. This was proof of the greatest psychological skill. "Under any other circumstances," Sylvie Trémillon notes, "such a vague gesture in the name of liberation would have invited harsh repression that might well have ended in a bloodbath. In this case nothing of the sort occurred: mythological culture, superstition, triumphed over political will."[1]

Faced with the pharaoh's intransigence, the god of the Hebrews inflicted on all of Egypt, around 1250 B.C., a series of scourges announced one after another by Moses and designated in the Bible by the term *oth*, traditionally translated as "plague." But the Hebrew word may also mean "blow" or "letter," and so be understood as a "threatening message."[2] The account of this episode has come down to us through chapters 7–12 of the book of Exodus, composed two centuries later. The question arises whether a rational explanation for each of the ten plagues can be derived from the medical, entomological, geographical, astronomical, and meteorological information available to us.

Water Turned to Blood

In the first instance, at the command of Moses, Aaron transformed the waters of the Nile into blood. The pharaoh did not react to this scourge, which his magicians are said to have succeeded in reproducing. Two consequences of this remarkable act are of particular interest: water was made unfit to drink, and fish died in great numbers.

Four explanations of these phenomena have been advanced. The most familiar one is that the floodwaters of the Nile swept away the earth of the banks of its upper course, and that the ochre (iron oxides) in the soil stained the water red. Moses, an excellent astronomer and meteorologist, could easily have predicted this periodic phenomenon. A second hypothesis involves a fresh outbreak of urinary schistosomiasis causing hematuria (blood in the urine). But this condition, as we have seen, was endemic—so how to explain the fear it aroused in the Egyptian people? Trémillon has suggested that the outbreak might have occurred after the floods had receded, when the Nile was at its lowest level and its current substantially slowed, with the result that widespread hematuria arising from a massive parasitic infestation of the population tinted stagnant pools of water in addition to the river's waters: "The Egyptians would surely have been surprised," she remarks, "to see the water turn red so late in the year."[3]

A third, quite interesting, proposal made by Louis Fage has the advantage of accounting for several of the other plagues as well. Fage argued that the red color of the Nile may have been caused by a sudden proliferation of unicellular plantlike marine organisms belonging to the order of dinoflagellates. This hypothesis depends on the assumption that an abrupt rise in the waters of the Nile would have produced a considerable increase in the number of these microorganisms by providing the nutritive salts (nitrates, iron, phosphates) necessary to their metabolism. Two pieces of evidence may be cited in favor of the proposition that dinoflagellates played an important role in this first plague: first, they contain a bright red photoreceptor stigma that imparts a reddish fluorescence to the water's surface; second, they secrete toxins that are fatal to most fish that come into contact with them.[4]

The fourth hypothesis, independently proposed by two geologists, William Ryan and Gilles Lericolais, blames a volcanic eruption on the island of Thera (also known as Santorin or Santorini) in the south Aegean Sea during the seventeenth century B.C. In the two days that its eruption probably lasted, the volcano threw up some thirty cubic kilometers of ash and lava. The eruption would have produced a tidal wave whose effects may have been felt as far away as the Egyptian coast. According to Lericolais, the red color of the Nile was caused by ignimbrite (rock formed by the accumulation of acid lava debris, such as rhyolite) carried by the storm surge. Ryan, by contrast, stresses the high sulfuric acid content of the volcanic particles, which may have oxidized the ferrous stone of the riverbed, giving a rust-colored sheen to the water.[5]

Frogs

Seven days later Aaron caused Egypt to be invaded by a multitude of frogs. This plague has given rise to a variety of interpretations, not least because frogs, along with snakes, occupy a major place in Egyptian cosmogony as the first inhabitants of the earth.

Two scientific explanations for their proliferation have been suggested. The first, proposed by Jean Lescure, is that a sudden increase in humidity following a prolonged dry spell in the Egyptian semi-desert triggered a massive migration of frogs searching for water. The second assumes that the digging of new wells, owing to the pollution of the Nile caused by the first plague, modified the local ecosystem in relevant ways. Frogs usually hibernate during the winter, and then during their period of sexual activity in the spring seek out ponds in which to lay and fertilize eggs. With the creation of additional water sources, frogs would have benefited from an environment that now favored their multiplication. Females can be extremely prolific, each laying as many as a thousand eggs.[6]

Mosquitoes

The plague of mosquitoes, which Egyptian magicians were unable to reproduce, must also have been connected with an increase in the number of water sources following the poisoning of the Nile. Interestingly, the pharaoh did not react in this case, perhaps because such infestations were not uncommon in the many hot, humid, and marshy places found in Egypt.[7]

Flies

The swarms of flies that invaded the houses of the Egyptians, while sparing those of the Hebrews, were probably another natural phenomenon associated with the seasonal rise in the waters of the Nile and intensified by the putrefaction of dead frogs.

It should be emphasized that the flies and mosquitoes mentioned in the third and fourth plagues were likely to have transmitted a certain number of human and animal diseases. Female *Anopheles* are vectors for malaria; *Culex pipiens* for Bancroft's filariasis; *Aedes aegypti* for dengue and yellow fever; and bloodsucking flies for pathogenic agents in humans. The common housefly is a carrier of many germs, such as *Bacillus anthracis*, responsible for anthrax; *Chlamydia trachomatis*, responsible for the eye disease trachoma; and *Shigella dysenteriae*, which causes bacillary dysentery.

Livestock Pest

The fifth plague was a disease that devastated all the herds of livestock (bovines, ovines, equids) belonging to the Egyptians while sparing those of the Hebrews. It is difficult to establish a definitive diagnosis in the absence of a precise description of symptoms. Four afflictions may nonetheless be imagined: rinderpest (cattle plague), foot-and-mouth disease, Rift Valley fever, and above all anthrax—the latter by virtue of its enzootic character, the type of animal affected, and the grave prognosis for this disease.

Sores

After Moses threw handfuls of ashes into the air came the sixth plague: the sky was plunged into darkness and the bodies of both the Egyptians and their animals were covered with pustules and ulcers. Several underlying conditions have been associated with these symptoms, in particular smallpox (by Ange Pierre Leca and Amin Gemayel). The strongest argument on behalf of this diagnosis is the finding of traces of smallpox in the mummy of Rameses II, evidence that this disease existed in Egypt during the period when the ten plagues occurred. Neither leishmaniasis nor furuncular myiasis can be ruled out, however, as they both cause sores on the skin. The earlier proliferation of flies, which are known to be responsible for these two parasitic diseases, counts in their favor as well. The fact that the Hebrews were not victims of this condition might be a consequence of preventive measures that required them to quarantine anyone with a lesion of the skin.[8]

Hail

Pointing his rod toward the sky, Moses next brought forth thunder and hail, striking fear into the Egyptians while sparing the Hebrews and their herds.

Two hypotheses have been proposed. The first rests on a meteorological phenomenon that is very rare in Egypt but has been observed on several occasions, in particular in May 1945 by the Egyptologist Pierre Montet, who witnessed a rain of walnut-sized hail that, according to his account, crushed the crops in the fields in five minutes, injuring people and animals alike.[9] One wonders whether such an event might not have occurred when Moses confronted the pharaoh.

A second hypothesis, proposed by Jean-François Royer, a climatologist at Météo-France, involves the possibility that particulate matter emitted by the Santorini volcano helped to create the condensation nuclei necessary to cause rain or hail. The hail may in fact have consisted of both ice and accreted ashes, or lapilli.[10]

Locusts

The violent hail of the seventh plague may also have favored the hatching and proliferation of swarms of locusts *(Locusta migratoria)*. During their migratory period locusts are capable of traveling large distances, as much as 2,500 miles in two months, and form "clouds" made up of thousands of insects that may cover as much as 350–400 square miles. The biblical invasion was carried by an east wind that probably came from the Middle East—a phenomenon that was particularly dreaded by the Egyptian peasants, who wore amulets inscribed with the image of the locust to protect themselves against it.[11]

Darkness

The ninth plague was rich in significance, for the pharaoh was considered the son of Ra, the sun god. The biblical account that for three days Egypt was plunged into darkness has suggested two possible explanations. The first posits the occurrence of a khamsin, a desert wind that blows several times a year and raises a cloud of dust and sand dense enough to block out daylight.

The second hypothesis refers back once more to the effects of a large cloud of particles emitted by the Santorini volcano. An identical phenomenon was recorded in 1991 after the eruption of Mount Pinatubo in the Philippines, which spewed some twenty megatons of sulfur dioxide into the atmosphere and covered Manila with the equivalent of 71 million truckloads of ash, forming a deposit 5 centimeters thick over more than 1,500 square miles and causing average global temperature to fall by several tenths of a degree for two winters.[12]

<hr>

Death of
the Firstborn

The most terrifying of all the scourges came in response to the massacre of Hebrew children with the Lord's promise to Moses and Aaron to "smite all the firstborn in the land of Egypt, both man and beast." Even allowing for the undoubtedly high incidence of infant mortality during the New Kingdom, a lethal epidemic that affected both children and animals would appear to have been an exceptional event. Several explanations have been advanced.

The biblical account has usually been understood to involve plague. This diagnosis cannot be formally established, however, since the term "plague" is often improperly used to cover a number of extremely serious diseases that raged during antiquity. The celebrated plague of Athens in 331 B.C., for example, was more probably an epidemic of typhus. Bubonic plague seems to have been rife in Egypt only after the Muslim conquest in the seventh century A.D.[13]

Acute anterior poliomyelitis (polio) and measles have also been proposed as candidates, but neither of these viral infections affects animals. Two parasitic diseases have been suspected with greater justification: visceral leishmaniasis, which is transmitted by very small bloodsucking sand flies of the genus *Phlebotomus;* and, above all, malaria.[14] The Santorini volcano is once again a possibility, though in this case not as an immediate cause of the epidemic, but rather through its indirect effects. Dr. Rayana Bu-Hakah of the World Health Organization has pointed out that a natural catastrophe such as the eruption of a volcano forces people to move and regroup. A lack of clean water frequently leads to a deterioration in public hygiene, and diseases such as cholera are apt to appear extremely quickly, sometimes within two days of such an eruption.[15]

The fact of the matter is that we are not able, on the basis of the information now available to us, to determine the exact nature of the tenth plague, which caused the death of the pharaoh's eldest son.[16] In the aftermath of this calamity the bereaved pharaoh permitted the Hebrews to leave, acknowledging that the power of the god of Israel surpassed his own. Nonetheless he quickly regretted his weakness and the loss of so many slaves, and pursued the departing Hebrews at the head of an army.

In the biblical account of the parting of the Red Sea, immortalized in the cinema by Cecil B. DeMille, the Hebrews were able to escape from Egypt before the pharaoh and his men were swallowed up by the resurgent waters. This scene, no less than the ten plagues of Egypt themselves, has been the object of many interpretations, in this case meteorological. The most appealing one comes from Doron Nof and Nathan Paldor, who have used a computer model of the basin of the Red Sea to show that moderate wind blowing for several hours could have rendered this expanse of shallow water passable, pushing back the waters up to a height of eight feet. A simple change in the direction of the wind would have been enough to cause this wall of water to collapse.[17]

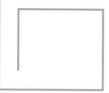

Chronology of Ancient Egypt

The table that follows is based upon the chronology officially accepted by the department of Egyptian antiquities at the Louvre. It lists only the most important rulers. The dates given are sometimes approximate and may slightly differ from those found in other works.

Late Predynastic Period

Naqada I Period	3800–3500 B.C.
Naqada II Period	3500–3300 B.C.
Naqada III Period	3300–3100 B.C.

Unification of Egypt by the legendary king Narmer (or by the 1st Dynasty ruler Menes).

Early Dynastic Period

1st Dynasty	3100–2900 B.C.
2nd Dynasty	2900–2700 B.C.

Old Kingdom

3rd Dynasty	2700–2620 B.C.
Djoser (2680–2650)	
4th Dynasty	2620–2500 B.C.
Sneferu (2620–2590)	
Khufu [Cheops] (2590–2565)	
Djedefra (2565–2558)	
Khafra [Chephren] (2558–2533)	
Menkaura [Mycerinus] (2533–2503)	
5th Dynasty	2500–2350 B.C.
Sahura (2492–2480)	
Neferirkara (2480–2470)	

Nyuserra (2453–2420)
Unas (2380–2350)
6th Dynasty   2350–2190 B.C.
   Pepy I (2320–2290)
   Pepy II (2270–2190)

Fragmentation of power and division of the country.

First Intermediate Period
7th Dynasty (according to Menethus, "Seventy kings in seventy days")
8th Dynasty   2190–2150 B.C.
9th Dynasty   2150–2100 B.C.
10th Dynasty   2100–2050 B.C.
11th Dynasty   2106–2033 B.C.

Reunification of the country about 2033 B.C., ushering in the Middle Kingdom under the rule of the last three pharaohs of the 11th Dynasty.

Middle Kingdom
11th Dynasty   2033–1963 B.C.
12th Dynasty   1963–1786 B.C.
   Amenemhat I (1963–1934)
   Senusret I (1934–1898)
   Amenemhat II (1898–1866)
   Senusret II (1866–1862)
   Senusret III (1862–1843)
   Amenemhat III (1843–1798)
13th Dynasty   1786–1710 B.C.
14th Dynasty   1710–1650 B.C.

Fragmentation of power about 1650 B.C., followed by the occupation of the
country by the Hyksos.

Second Intermediate Period
15th Dynasty (Hyksos)   1650–1550 B.C.
16th Dynasty   1650–1580 B.C.
17th Dynasty   1580–1550 B.C.

New Kingdom
18th Dynasty   1550–1295 B.C.
   Ahmose I (1550–1525)
   Amenhotep I (1525–1504)

Thutmose I (1504–1492)
Thutmose II (1492–1479)
Thutmose III (1479–1425)
Queen Hatshepsut (1479–1457)
Amenhotep II (1425–1401)
Thutmose IV (1401–1391)
Amenhotep III (1391–1353)
Amenhotep IV/Akhenaten (1353–1337)
Neferneferuaten [Smenkhkara] (1338–1336)
Tutankhamun (1336–1327)
Ay (1327–1323)
Horemheb (1323–1295)

Ramessid Period

19th Dynasty	1295–1186 B.C.
Rameses I (1295–1294)	
Sety I (1294–1279)	
Rameses II (1279–1213)	
Merenptah (1213–1203)	
Sety II (1200–1194)	
20th Dynasty	1186–1069 B.C.
Rameses III (1184–1153)	

Third Intermediate Period

21st Dynasty	1069–945 B.C.
22nd Dynasty	945–715 B.C.
23rd Dynasty (Libyan)	818–715 B.C.
24th Dynasty (Libyan)	727–715 B.C.
25th Dynasty	780–656 B.C.

Period of Ethiopian (or Kushite) domination
Piy (747–716)

Late Period

26th Dynasty	664–525 B.C.
27th Dynasty	525–404 B.C.
1st Persian Period	
28th Dynasty	404–399 B.C.
29th Dynasty	398–379 B.C.
30th Dynasty	378–341 B.C.
2nd Persian Period	340–332 B.C.

Ptolemaic Period   332–30 B.C.

Alexander the Great (332–323)
Ptolemy I–Ptolemy XII (305–51)
Cleopatra VII (51–30)

Roman Period   30 B.C.–A.D. 395

Egypt annexed by Augustus Caesar in 30 B.C. as a Roman province.
Arab conquest in A.D. 641.

Notes

Introduction

1. Lichtenthaeler, *Histoire de la médecine.*
2. Champdor, *Le livre des morts.* Spaeth, "Pneumologie et cancérologie dans la médecine de l'Égypte à travers les écrits médicaux, l'art et les données de la paléopathologie." Jean Vercoutter, *À la recherche de l'Égypte oubliée.*
3. Ackerknecht, "Paleopathology," quoted in Spaeth, "Pneumologie et cancérologie," 14.

1. The Medical Profession

1. Boulu, "Le médecin dans la civilisation de l'Égypte pharaonique," 52. [Serqet, often referred to by her Greek name, Selkis, was represented sometimes with the head of a scorpion, sometimes as a scorpion with the head of a woman.—Trans.]
2. Rachet, *Dictionnaire de la civilisation égyptienne;* see also Ritner, "Magic in Medicine." Posener, Sauneron, and Yoyotte, *Dictionnaire de la civilisation égyptienne,* 251.
3. Lucian of Samosata, "The Syrian Goddess," 2. The first representations of divinities date from the Predynastic Period. Each tribe living in the Nile Valley had its own god, represented by an animal. In time these depictions came to assume a human form. The Egyptian pantheon was very large and included gods responsible for vital functions (fertility, birth, the Nile, harvests, and so on), funerary gods, innumerable local gods, some of whom later became gods of the Egyptian people generally, and cosmogonic gods, responsible for the creation of the world.

4. Lexa, *La magie dans l'Égypte antique*. Hornung, *L'esprit au temps des pharaons*, 49. Rachet, *Dictionnaire*, 153. Daumas, *La civilisation de l'Égypte pharaonique*, 547; see also Ritner, "Medicine."

5. Leca, *La médecine égyptienne au temps des pharaons*, 59. Hennequin, "Santé et hygiène de l'enfant dans l'Égypte ancienne," 49. Woodward, "Religion and Medicine."

6. Posener, Sauneron, and Yoyotte, *Dictionnaire*, 27. Ey, *Naissance de la médecine*, 230. Lichtenthaeler, *Histoire de la médecine*, 85. In the preceding ("primitive-magical") phase, typical of tribal societies, disease was thought to be caused by external agents that justified treatment by a sha-man, or "medicine man," in order "to extract and eliminate the causal factor." A third phase in the Western tradition is characterized by "a positive medical doctrine based on scientific analysis," as in the case of Hippocrates; see Jouanna, *Hippocrates*, 141–176.

7. Spaeth, "Pneumologie et cancérologie dans la médecine de l'Égypte," 15. Lefebvre, *Essai sur la médecine égyptienne de l'époque pharaonique*, 9.

8. Leca, *La médecine égyptienne*, 104.

9. Boulu, "Le médecin," 13. "Le médecin de pharaon," *Sciences et avenir*.

10. Picard, "La médecine magique dans l'Égypte ancienne," 37. Driesch, "Is There a Veterinary Papyrus of Kahun?"

11. Boulu, "Le médecin," 54. Jonckheere, *Les médecins de l'Égypte pharaonique*, 131. An inscription on the tomb of Petosiris, overseer of the priests of Sekhmet, reads: "Your herd is numerous in the stable thanks to the science of the priests of Sekhmet."

12. Jonckheere, "La place du prêtre de Sekhmet dans le corps médical de l'ancienne Égypte." Spaeth, "Pneumologie et cancérologie," 35.

13. Maspero, *Études de mythologie et d'archéologie égyptienne*, 1: 302. For Greek practitioners see the discussion of Asclepiad priests and physicians in Jouanna, *Hippocrates*, 195–203. Boulu, "Le médecin," 52. Picard, "La médecine magique," 85.

14. Boulu, "Le médecin," 55. Another Ptahhotep of the same period is identified by his tomb inscription as "*wab*-priest of Sekhmet, inspector of physicians, Wenennefer." Moreover, a stele of the Middle Kingdom dating from the reign of Amenemhat III describes one Nedjemu-seneb as "overseer of the priests of Sekhmet and chief of physicians." See Boulu, "Le médecin," 54–55.

15. Quotation from Picard, "La médecine magique," 87. Koenig, *Magie et magiciens dans l'Égypte ancienne*, 20–22.

16. Gardiner, "Professional Magicians in Ancient Egypt." Boulu, "Le médecin," 57. Frédérique von Känel distinguishes between *sa Serqet* and *kherep Serqet*, translating the former term as "protector of Serqet," an ep-

ithet meant to stress the ritualistic aspect of exorcism, by contrast with the medical role implied by the latter term. See *Les prêtres-ouâb de Sekhmet et les conjurateurs de Serket,* 284.

17. This text, found on a healing statue, is cited in Boulu, "Le médecin," 56.
18. Ibid. [Irenakhty is not to be confused with another practitioner of the same name who was active some 150 years later: see Nunn's list of known doctors in *Ancient Egyptian Medicine,* 211–214; also Nunn's extensive compendium of medical hieroglyphs.—Trans.]
19. Jonckheere, "À la recherche du chirurgien égyptien." [Nunn, who gives the term as *sahemem,* construes it as the name of a cauterizing treatment and says that it cannot at present be translated. But other authorities, including Ebbell and Ghalioungui, agree with Jonckheere that it refers to a practitioner expert in the use of heated instruments *(hemem).* Bardinet concurs.—Trans.]
20. Herodotus 2.84, from *The Histories,* trans. Sélincourt, 114 (hereafter referred to as Sélincourt). [The reference to "innumerable doctors" may have been influenced, as Sélincourt observes, by Homer's claim that the Egyptians are descended from the physician of the gods, Paeëon.—Trans.]
21. Pliny the Elder, *Natural History* 26.3 (Loeb, 7:266–267). Boulu cites two such specialists who practiced during the Old Kingdom, Wa and Nefertjes, both styled "doctor of the eyes" and attached to the royal palace, and, during the First Intermediate Period, Irenakhty. During the New Kingdom he mentions Huy, administrator and chief of the physicians of the eyes of the palace, and, in the Late Period, another Wa and Padi. See Boulu, "Le médecin," 61. [Here, as elsewhere, anglicized versions of physicians' names are given instead of their French spellings.—Trans.]
22. Lefebvre, *Essai sur la médecine égyptienne,* 59. Nickol et al., "An Examination of the Dental State of an Egyptian Mummy by Means of Computer Tomography." Boulu, "Le médecin," 63. The names of two other dentists attached to the royal palace bearing the title *wer ibhy per aa* ("chief dentist of the palace") are known. Paul Ghalioungui argues in *La médecine des pharaons* that the fact that neither of the two *ibhy* was a physician, unlike the "chief dentist," suggests that they may have held the position of technical assistant or else have been students.
23. Viso and Uriach, "The 'Guardians of the Anus' and Their Practice." [Other translations of this term include "herdsmen" and "shepherds" of the anus.—Trans.]
24. Herodotus 2.77, Sélincourt, 113. Diodorus Siculus 1.82 (Loeb, 1:280–281). Ghalioungui compares these physicians to the Greek *iatroklystes;* see *La médecine des pharaons,* 85.
25. Spaeth, "Pneumologie et cancérologie," 62.

26. Jonckheere, "Le cadre professionel et administratif des médecins égyptiens." Leca, *La médecine égyptienne,* 106.

27. Meeks, "Notes de lexicographies."

28. Boulu, "Le médecin," 69, 68. Jonckheere, *Les médecins de l'Égypte pharaonique.*

29. Ghalioungui, *La médecine des pharaons,* 44. Leca, *La médecine égyptienne,* 108.

30. Godron, "Notes sur l'histoire de la médecine et l'occupation perse en Égypte." Boulu, "Le médecin," 69. Grapow, von Deines, and Westendorf, *Grundriss der Medizin der alten Ägypter,* 3:97.

31. The account that follows is at odds with the one given by Nunn in *Ancient Egyptian Medicine,* 116–120. And indeed in many places where the Egyptian names used in different periods are lacking, it is impossible even to reconcile English and French translations of the titles themselves, which in any case remain subject to considerable uncertainty. On physicians' identities and titles see also Ghalioungui, *The Physicians of Pharaonic Egypt.—* Trans.

32. Bardinet, "Les médecins dans la société égyptienne à l'époque des pharaons."

33. Ibid.

34. Picard, "La médecine magique," 37. Note, for example, the combination of titles borne by Nesemnaw (4th–5th Dynasties) and by Nyankhkhnum (6th Dynasty), who were styled, respectively, chief of physicians (an extrapalatine title) and physician of the palace.

35. We know the names of a certain number of physicians who held the post of chief physician *(wer swnw),* among them Nyankhsekhmet, personal physician to King Sahura, who lived around 2400 B.C. during the 5th Dynasty, and Khuy, about a century later under the reigns of Teti and Pepy I in the 6th Dynasty.

36. See Bardinet, "Les médecins."

37. Ibid.

38. Two chief physicians to the king *(wer swnw n nesu)* are now known, in particular a certain Heryshefnakht under the 12th Dynasty.

39. Thus, for example, Bakenkhonsu, who worked in Thebes during the Third Intermediate Period, bore the title of chief physician to the Lord of the Two Lands.

40. Boulu, "Le médecin," 182. Helck, "Eine Briefsammlung aus der Verwaltung des Amuntemples."

41. Boulu, "Le médecin," 173.

42. Quoted in ibid., 166.

43. Bardinet, *Les papyrus médicaux de l'Égypte pharaonique,* 83. [The "Book

of the Heart" is sometimes called "The Physician's Secret," after its opening lines (in Ebbell's translation): "The beginning of the physician's secret:
knowledge of the heart's movement and knowledge of the heart."—
Trans.]

44. Nanetti, "Ricerche sui medici e sulla medecina nei papiri." Boulu, "Le
médecin," 164.

45. Boulu, "Le médecin," 162. Diodorus Siculus 1.82 (Loeb, 1:280–281).

46. Černý, "Quelques ostracas hiératiques inédits de Thèbes au musée du
Caire." Boulu, "Le médecin," 158; a *khar* amounted to roughly 76 liters
(about 20 gallons). Janssen, *Commodity Prices from the Ramessid Period,*
460.

47. Papyrus Turin 2071, quoted in Jonckheere, *Les médecins de l'Égypte
pharaonique,* 85. Edgerton, "The Strikes in Rameses III's Twenty-Ninth
Year," 142–143. A fragment of the Vatican papyrus describes payments
made to several individuals, one of them a physician of the necropolis
who is mentioned in the Turin Canon, which dates from the twenty-ninth
year of the reign of Rameses III. Several papyri of the Ptolemaic period
also mention the payment of a tax by Greek military settlers to physicians—but this is a late piece of evidence.

48. Picard, "La médecine magique," 41. Boulu, "Le médecin," 156.

49. Jonckheere, *Les médecins de l'Égypte pharaonique.*

2. Training and Practice

1. Martinez, *Égypte,* 94. [Whatever the figure for Deir el-Medina, it would
have been considerably higher than the one for the New Kingdom population as a whole.—Trans.]

2. Brunner, "L'éducation en ancienne Égypte." Martinez, *Égypte.* Lefebvre,
Essai sur la médecine égyptienne de l'époque pharaonique.

3. Diodorus Siculus 1.81 (Loeb, 1:278–279), 1.74 (Loeb, 1:256–257). Nunn,
Ancient Egyptian Medicine, 130.

4. Boulu, "Le médecin dans la civilisation de l'Égypte pharaonique," 42.
Martinez, *Égypte,* 95. Quotation from *The Maxims of Ptahhotep,* an important Old Kingdom literary work, in Sarazin, "La pathologie cardio-
vasculaire dans l'Égypte ancienne."

5. Posener quoted in Picard, "La médecine magique dans l'Égypte ancienne,"
33.

6. Gardiner, "The House of Life." Moreover, during the Late Period, when
hieroglyphic writing was exclusively a priestly practice, hieroglyphs were
called "the writings of the house of life." See Gunn, "Interpreters of
Dreams in Ancient Egypt."

7. Volten, *Demotische Traumdeutung*, 20. Lefebvre, *Essai sur la médecine égyptienne.*

8. Martinez, *Égypte.* Lefebvre, *Essai sur la médecine égyptienne.* Gardiner, "House of Life," 160.

9. Boulu, "Le médecin," 46. This inscription is preserved today in the Vatican Museum: see Leca, *La médecine égyptienne au temps des pharaons,* 123.

10. Quoted in Picard, "La médecine magique," 34–36.

11. Boulu, "Le médecin," 46. Gardiner, "House of Life."

12. Boulu, "Le médecin," 47.

13. Von Känel, *Les prêtres-ouâb de Sekhmet et les conjurateurs de Serket.* Jonckheere, "Le 'préparateur de remèdes' dans l'organisation de la pharmacie égyptienne," quoted in Boulu, "Le médecin," 47.

14. Lefebvre, *Essai sur la médecine égyptienne,* 22. [Here I adopt Bardinet's literal translation of this phrase in Edwin Smith 20. Breasted says simply: "If thou ask of him concerning his malady . . ."—Trans.]

15. Regarding the different senses of *ib* see Chapter 7, note 15.—Trans.

16. Edwin Smith 1, quoted in Lethor, "Du coeur et des vaisseaux dans l'Égypte ancienne," 65. [Breasted points out that the word for "examining" literally means "measuring."—Trans.] Gispen, "Measuring the Patient in Ancient Egyptian Medical Texts." Ebbell, *The Papyrus Ebers,* 21. Breasted, *The Edwin Smith Surgical Papyrus,* 1:38.

17. Lethor, "Du coeur et des vaisseaux," 65. Caton, "The Medicine and the Medicine God of the Egyptians."

18. Spaeth, "Pneumologie et cancérologie dans la médecine de l'Égypte," 93. Atta, "Edwin Smith Surgical Papyrus."

19. Quotation from Picard, "La médecine magique," 19. Koenig, "Religion and Medicine I."

20. Diodorus Siculus 1.82 (Loeb, 1:280–283). Aristotle, *Politics,* book 3, 1286a (Loeb, 21:256–257).

21. Bontemps, "La médecine en Égypte pharaonique," 92. Ghalioungui, *La médecine des pharaons,* 18. Hennequin, "Santé et hygiène de l'enfant dans l'Égypte ancienne," 50.

22. Ghalioungui, *La médecine des pharaons,* 18. Hennequin, "Santé et hygiène de l'enfant," 50.

23. See the discussion of Ebers 1–3 in Bardinet, *Les papyrus médicaux de l'Égypte pharaonique,* 39–48.

24. Ebers 250 gives a recipe for treating migraine, "the aches that are on one side of the head." The Egyptian term *ges-tep,* or "half-head," was taken over by the Greeks as *hemikrania,* the source of the English word for this malady.—Trans.

25. Picard, "La médecine magique," 63.
26. Koenig, *Magie et magiciens dans l'Égypte ancienne,* 132. Picard, "La médecine magique," 63.
27. Riad, *La médecine au temps des pharaons,* 244. Graffito quoted in Hennequin, "Santé et hygiène de l'enfant," 58.
28. Daumas, "Le sanatorium de Dendera." Hennequin, "Santé et hygiène de l'enfant," 59.
29. Riad, *La médecine au temps des pharaons,* 249.
30. Thus notations such as 1/16 and 1/32 are to be read as so many parts of a *heqat.*—Trans.
31. Nunn, *Ancient Egyptian Medicine,* 140–141. [The plural form *henu* is used by Nunn and other authors; strictly speaking it is the singular *hin* that is meant.—Trans.]
32. Bowman, "Drugs Ancient and Modern."
33. Zumla and Lulat, "Honey." The use, for example, of fecal matter in treating burns on the second day, recommended in Ebers 482, seems unwise today.
34. Boulu, "Le médecin," 73. Nunn, who claims there is no known Egyptian word for pharmacist, overlooks the fact that this was one of the titles of the 5th Dynasty physician Iry; see Bardinet, *Dents et mâchoires,* 235.
35. The term "myrrh" in this title stands for the entire pharmacopoeia, the guardian of which was also responsible for preparing the remedies ordered by the *swnw.* See Leca, *La médecine égyptienne,* 120.
36. Feldman and Goodrich, "The Edwin Smith Surgical Papyrus."
37. Nunn and Andrew, "Egyptian Antiquities at the Royal College of Surgeons of England." Hamarneh, "Excavated Surgical Instruments from Old Cairo, Egypt."
38. Lucas and Harris, *Ancient Egyptian Materials and Industries,* 142–146.
39. Edwin Smith 11 is a typical example. See Breasted, *Edwin Smith Surgical Papyrus,* 1:8.
40. The term "lint" *(ftt)* refers here to "some kind of vegetable tissue obtained from a plant called . . . *dby·t*" having absorbent properties and used, in combination with a honey ointment, for both external application and insertion in bodily orifices. See ibid., 1:101.—Trans.
41. Ibid., 1:316. [Breasted's opinion on this, as on almost all other technical questions of medicine, in which he had no training, was due to the eminent surgeon Dr. Arno B. Luckhardt of the University of Chicago. See Breasted's acknowledgment of Luckhardt's assistance, page xix.—Trans.]
42. Menard, "Les techniques chirurgicales dans l'antiquité égyptienne," 100.
43. Breasted, *Edwin Smith Surgical Papyrus,* 1:8. Jonckheere, "À la recherche du chirurgien égyptien."

44. Lefebvre, *Essai sur la médecine égyptienne*. See cases 2, 9, 10, and 47 in the Edwin Smith papyrus.

45. Lucas and Harris, *Ancient Egyptian Materials and Industries*, 1–9, 316–324.

46. Lefebvre, *Essai sur la médecine égyptienne*. Petrie, *Tools and Weapons*.

47. Breasted, *Edwin Smith Surgical Papyrus*, 1:264–265.

48. Dioscorides, *De simplicibus medicinis*, 5.158. ["It is said that this being beaten small, and smeared upon the places that shall be cut, or burnt, doth bring in them a stupid senselessness, without danger": see the 1655 English translation by John Goodyer of the Latin version of this treatise, *De materia medica*, published as *The Greek Herbal of Dioscorides*, 655.—Trans.]

49. Riad, *La médecine au temps des pharaons*, 249. Nunn, *Ancient Egyptian Medicine*, 169. Baslez, "Les poisons dans l'antiquité égyptienne."

3. Mummification

1. Hennequin, "Santé et hygiène de l'enfant dans l'Égypte ancienne," 5.

2. Wiltse and Pait, "Herophilus of Alexandria." See also von Staden, *Herophilus*, 139–154. Lethor, "Du coeur et des vaisseaux dans l'Égypte ancienne," 60.

3. Lefebvre, *Essai sur la médecine égyptienne de l'époque pharaonique*. Dollfus, "Les connaissances neurologiques des anciens égyptiens," 2.

4. Sauneron, "Une conception anatomique tardive."

5. Assmann, *Images et rites de la mort dans l'Égypte ancienne*. On the parts of the individual see Redford, ed., *Oxford Encyclopedia of Ancient Egypt*, 3:237–238.

6. Redford, ed., *The Ancient Gods Speak*, xvi–xvii, 169–170, 331–332. Rachet, *Dictionnaire de la civilisation égyptienne*, 171.

7. Dunand and Lichtenberg, *Les momies et la mort en Égypte*. See also David, "Mummification."

8. Koller et al., "Embalming Was Used in Old Kingdom." Goyon and Josset, *Un corps pour l'éternité*, 142.

9. Dunand and Lichtenberg, *Les momies et la mort*. Brier and Wade, "The Use of Natron in Egyptian Mummification."

10. Millo, "La mort chez les Égyptiens," 94.

11. Assmann, *Images et rites de la mort*.

12. The title is also often given as *hery sstaw*, or one with authority over the mysteries.

13. Bucaille, *Les momies des pharaons et la médecine*, 247.

14. Sluglett, "Mummification in Ancient Egypt."

15. Reyman, "Les momies égyptiennes." Salem and Eknoyan, "The Kidney in Ancient Egyptian Medicine."
16. Millo, "La mort chez les Égyptiens," 98. Herodotus 2.86. Diodorus Siculus 1.91.
17. Its duration was also controversial among ancient commentators: according to Genesis 50:3, forty days were required for embalming. Nonetheless, despite variations, seventy days seems to have been the most usual period; see Lucas and Harris, *Ancient Egyptian Materials and Industries,* 299.—Trans.
18. Bucaille, *Les momies des pharaons,* 247.
19. Herodotus 2.87–88.

4. The Modern Study of Mummies

1. Morice, "La gynécologie et l'obstétrique en Égypte pharaonique," 13. Henrion, "L'athérosclérose dans l'Égypte ancienne," 95.
2. Granville, "An Essay on Egyptian Mummies with Observations on the Art of Embalming among the Ancient Egyptians."
3. Cockburn et al., "Autopsy of an Egyptian Mummy." Balout et al., *La momie de Ramsès II,* 9.
4. David, "Mummification." Thorwald, *Histoire de la médecine dans l'antiquité,* 33. Fodor, Malott, and King, "The Radiographic Investigation of Two Egyptian Mummies"; also Bloomfield, "Radiology of Egyptian Mummy."
5. Riad, *La médecine au temps des pharaons,* 181. Moodie, *Roentgenologic Studies of Egyptian and Peruvian Mummies.* Gray, "Radiography of Ancient Egyptian Mummies."
6. Brothwell and Sandison, *Diseases in Antiquity,* 521–523. Faure and Bucaille, "Intérêt actuel de l'étude radiologique des momies pharaoniques." Dunand and Lichtenberg, *Les momies et la mort en Égypte,* 44.
7. Thekkaniyil, Bishara, and James, "Dental and Skeletal Findings on an Ancient Egyptian Mummy." De Bidart, "Momification et paléopathologie des momies de l'Égypte ancienne," 68.
8. Dunand and Lichtenberg, *Les momies et la mort,* 160.
9. The unembalmed and naturally preserved mummy of a weaver from the New Kingdom called Nakht (known also as ROM 1) and the mummy of Rameses II have been subjected to this technique: see Iles, "Autopsy of an Egyptian Mummy."
10. De Bidart, "Momification et paléopathologie," 68.
11. Harwood-Nash, "Computed Tomography of Ancient Egyptian

Mummies." Pahl, "Possibilities, Limitations, and Prospects of Computed Tomography as a Non-Invasive Method of Mummy Studies." Falke et al., "Computed Tomography of an Ancient Egyptian." Marx and D'Auria, "CT Examination of Eleven Egyptian Mummies."

12. Notman, "Ancient Scannings."

13. Marx and D'Auria, "Three-Dimensional CT Reconstructions of an Ancient Human Egyptian Mummy." Baldock et al., "3-D Reconstruction of an Ancient Egyptian Mummy Using X-Ray Computer Tomography." Hill, Macleod, and Watson, "Facial Reconstruction of a 3500-Year-Old Egyptian Mummy Using Axial Computed Tomography." Spaeth, "Pneumologie et cancérologie dans la médecine de l'Égypte," 146.

14. Piepenbrink et al., "Nuclear Magnetic Resonance Imaging of Mummified Corpses." For example, the results of nuclear magnetic resonance imaging performed in 1983 on the mummy of Lady Tashat, in the collections of the Minneapolis Institute of Art, were inconclusive: see Notman et al., "Modern Imaging and Endoscopic Biopsy Techniques in Egyptian Mummies."

15. Bontemps, "La médecine en Égypte pharaonique," 153. Gaafar, Abdel-Monem, and Elsheikh, "Nasal Endoscopy and CT Study of Pharaonic and Roman Mummies."

16. Bellouard, "Le dossier médical des pharaons de la Haute Époque," 95. Leca, *Les momies*, 204.

17. Leca, *Les momies*, 38.

18. Notman et al., "Modern Imaging and Endoscopic Biopsy Techniques." The first endoscopies were done on mummies in the Cairo Museum in 1975. See Manialawy and Meligny, "Endoscopic Examination of Egyptian Mummies."

19. Czermak cited in Riad, *La médecine*, 183. Shattock, "Minutes of a Meeting of the Pathological Section of the Royal Society of Medicine." Ruffer, *Studies in the Paleopathology of Egypt.* Sandison, "The Histological Examination of Mummified Material."

20. Reyman, Zimmerman, and Lewin, "Autopsy of an Egyptian Mummy."

21. Chapel, Mehregan, and Reyman, "Histologic Findings in Mummified Skin." Perrin et al., "Préservation des structures cutanées des momies égyptiennes."

22. Emery, *A Funerary Repast in an Egyptian Tomb of the Archaic Period.* David, "Disease in Egyptian Mummies."

23. De Bidart, "Momification et paléopathologie," 82.

24. Balout et al., *La momie de Ramsès II.* Birkett, Gummer, and Dawber, "Preservation of the Sub-Cellular Ultrastructure of Ancient Hair." Sandford and Kissling, "Multivariate Analysis of Elemental Hair Concen-

trations from a Medieval Nubian Population." David, "Disease in Egyptian Mummies." Moore, "Drugs in Ancient Populations."

25. Libby, *Radiocarbon Dating.*

26. Barraco, Reyman, and Cockburn, "Paleobiochemical Analysis of an Egyptian Mummy."

27. Henrion, "L'athérosclérose dans l'Égypte ancienne," 102. Connolly, "Kinship of Smenkhkare and Tutankhamon Demonstrated Serologically." Analysis of blood groups in mummies can be carried out not only on muscle tissue but also on hair, skin, and bone. See Boyd, "Les groupes sanguins chez les anciens égyptiens."

28. Ruffer, *Studies in the Paleopathology of Egypt.* Iles, "Autopsy of an Egyptian Mummy." Cockburn et al., "Autopsy of an Egyptian Mummy."

29. Miller et al., "Diagnosis of Plasmodium falciparum Infections in Mummies Using the Rapid Manual *Para*Sight™-F Test." [ELISA stands for Enzyme-Linked Immunosorbent Assay, a test for detecting exposure to an infectious agent in which an enzyme and its substrate (rather than a radioactive substance) are used to indicate the presence or absence of an antibody to the infection.—Trans.]

30. Barraco, "Paleobiochemistry." David, "Disease in Egyptian Mummies." Buckley, Stott, and Evershed, "Studies of Organic Residues from Ancient Egyptian Mummies Using High Temperature–Gas Chromotography–Mass Spectrometry."

31. Marota and Rollo, "Molecular Paleontology." Pääbo, "Preservation of DNA in Ancient Egyptian Mummies." Pääbo, "Molecular Cloning of Ancient Egyptian Mummy DNA." Miller et al., "Evidence of Myocardial Infarction in Mummified Human Tissue." Horem Kenisi, whose mummy was discovered at Deir el-Bahri in 1904–1905, was in charge of the teams of workers and artisans employed in the Valley of the Kings. Archaeological analysis of his mummy carried out in 1987 concluded that he died from a sudden fall, landing face down in the desert sand. See El-Mahdy, *Momies, mythes et magie,* 98–99.

32. Hedges and Sykes, "The Extraction and Isolation of DNA from Archeological Bone."

5. Mothers and Children

1. Desroches-Noblecourt, *La femme au temps des pharaons,* 221.

2. Grandet, *Hymnes de la religion d'Aton,* 49. Suys, *La sagesse d'Ani,* 59.

3. Rachet, *Dictionnaire de la civilisation égyptienne,* 156.

4. Martinez, *Égypte,* 92.

5. Carlsberg IV quoted in Stevens, "Gynaecology from Ancient Egypt."

6. Morice, "La gynécologie et l'obstétrique en Égypte pharaonique," 66. See also Jouanna, *Hippocrates*, 172. [An echo of the passage in *Sterile Women* can be found in another Hippocratic treatise, *Aphorisms* 5.59.—Trans.]

7. On a stele in the temple at Philae, dedicated in part to Khnum, one finds this inscription: "It is he [Khnum] who causes the seed of the king to be bound in the belly [of his wives]." See Sullivan, "Divine and Rational." [Khnum was believed to shape human beings, using a potter's wheel, and then to breathe life into them.—Trans.]

8. Martinez, *Égypte*, 92. [See note 15 below.—Trans.]

9. Sauneron, "À propos d'un prognostic de naissance." Grapow, von Deines, and Westendorf, *Grundriss der Medizin der alten Ägypter*. Thorwald, *Histoire de la médecine dans l'antiquité*, 100. Ghalioungui, Khalil, and Ammar, "On an Ancient Egyptian Method of Diagnosing Pregnancy and Determining Foetal Sex."

10. Sauneron, "Les dix mois précédents la naissance." Morice, Josset, and Colau, "Gynécologie et obstétrique dans l'ancienne Égypte." Morice, "La gynécologie et l'obstétrique," 70–71. Hippocrates, *Aphorisms* 5.37, 42, 52, 53 (Loeb, 4:166–173).

11. Berlin 196 (incorporating part of the text of Kahun 26).

12. Morice, Josset, and Colau, "Gynécologie et obstétrique." Guiart, "L'obstétrique dans l'ancienne Égypte." Hennequin, "Santé et hygiène de l'enfant dans l'Égypte ancienne," 100. Leca, *La médecine égyptienne au temps des pharaons*, 335.

13. Quoted in Desroches-Noblecourt, *La femme au temps des pharaons*, 464.

14. Leca, *La médecine égyptienne*, 334. Engelbach and Derry, "Mummification."

15. Bardinet follows the *Grundriss* in rendering the phrase *mut remetj* (literally "mother of mankind") as "placenta." Ebbell's reading of it as "womb" is supported by Nunn, however, who cites Weeks, "The Anatomical Knowledge of the Ancient Egyptians and the Representation of the Human Figure in Egyptian Art." See Nunn, *Ancient Egyptian Medicine*, 196.—Trans.

16. Hennequin, "Santé et hygiène de l'enfant," 90, 90n17.

17. Desroches-Noblecourt, *La femme au temps des pharaons*.

18. Posener, "L'attribution d'un nom à l'enfant."

19. Suys, *La sagesse d'Ani*, 8:1.

20. Janssen and Janssen, *Growing Up in Ancient Egypt*, 165.

21. Neither Bardinet nor Ebbell is sure of the proper translation of the last phrase (Ebbell says the woman's feet are crossed), but the sense is clear enough—namely, that the woman is weak.—Trans.

22. The tiger nut, or earth almond, is the rhizome or edible tuber of *Cyperus*

esculentus. On this and other points of medical botany see Mannliche, *An Ancient Egyptian Herbal.*—Trans.

23. This recipe, which was supposed to bring certain relief, also figures in Berlin 17.
24. Jonckheere, "Un chapître de pédiatrie égyptienne."
25. See, for example, Thutmose III at Deir el-Bahri temple.

6. Childhood and Adolescence

1. Romant, *La vie en Égypte aux temps antiques,* 13. Diodorus Siculus 1.80 (Loeb, 1:274–277).
2. The fact that this remedy is described at the end of a section (764–782) dealing with otological conditions suggests that the child in question may have suffered from an earache. Regarding the disputed identity of the *shepen*-plant, see Nunn, *Ancient Egyptian Medicine,* 154–155.
3. The form of urinary incontinence referred to seems to have been enuresis.
4. In French the tooth fairy is called a little mouse *(petite souris).*—Trans.
5. Smith and Dawson, *Egyptian Mummies.* Hennequin, "Santé et hygiène de l'enfant dans l'Égypte ancienne," 134.
6. Merkle et al., "Computed Tomographic Measurements of the Nasal Sinuses and Frontal Bone in Mummy Heads Artificially Deformed in Infancy." Willemot cited by Hennequin, "Santé et hygiène de l'enfant," 137. The study of mummies has yielded interesting information about irreversible lesions of the ear. Traces of manifestations of otitis and mastoiditis have been found on PUM II. Otoscopy of a mummy by W. F. Pirsig revealed multiple perforations of the eardrum, which Pirsig attributed to a tuberculosis of the middle ear. A CAT scan later confirmed the presence of benign and malign tumors in the maxillary sinuses.
7. Hennequin, "Santé et hygiène de l'enfant," 133, 137. Murray, "Fruits, Vegetables, Pulses, and Condiments."
8. Dioscorides, *De simplicibus medicinis* 2.35.
9. Winter, "L'hygiène dans l'Égypte pharaonique," 115. At least one physician is believed to have borne the title "overseer of fumigation for the palace": see Guest, "Ancient Egyptian Physicians."
10. Hennequin, "Santé et hygiène de l'enfant," 130. Belmondo, "Nosologie égyptienne," 32–69.
11. Dawson cited in Hennequin, "Santé et hygiène de l'enfant," 127. Grapow, von Deines, and Westendorf, *Grundriss der Medizin der alten Ägypter.* Bardinet, "Le mot *bââ,* dans les papyrus médicaux de l'Égypte pharaonique."
12. Herodotus says: "The Phoenicians and the Syrians of Palestine recognized

that they held this practice [circumcision] from the Egyptians" (2.104). Diodorus Siculus (2.32) and Strabo (6.4.17) believed that the Hebrews had brought the practice back from Egypt.

13. Bellouard, "Le dossier médical des pharaons de la Haute Époque," 48.

14. Grossman and Posner, "The Circumcision Controversy." Waszak, "The Historic Significance of Circumcision." Herodotus 2.37 (Sélincourt, 99).

15. Thorwald, *Histoire de la médecine dans l'antiquité,* 53. Nunn, *Ancient Egyptian Medicine,* 169. Herodotus 2.86. Ann Macy Roth has argued that this scene depicts an initiation ceremony for *hemka*-priests that involved shaving the pubis rather than circumcision: see Nunn, ibid., 170–171. Another scene, dating from the New Kingdom (about 1350 B.C.) and representing the circumcision of two children of Rameses II, was discovered in the northeast courtyard of the temple of Mont at Karnak: see Chabas, "De la circumcision chez les Égyptiens."

16. Quoted in Desroches-Noblecourt, *La femme au temps des pharaons,* 269. [The East African kingdom of Punt, first visited by Egyptian traders during the 5th Dynasty, was long a byword for mystery and exoticism.— Trans.]

17. A more poetic version of the entire text, due to Alan H. Gardiner, can be found in Glanville, *The Legacy of Egypt,* 77.—Trans.

18. Rachet, *Dictionnaire de la civilisation égyptienne,* 44–45.

19. Quoted in Desroches-Noblecourt, *La femme au temps des pharaons.*

20. Quoted in Erman, *La civilisation égyptienne,* 751.

21. Quoted in Bontemps, "La médecine en Égypte pharaonique," 22.

22. Quoted in ibid.

7. Old Age and Deformities

1. Anastasi III (4, 89), cited in Leca, *La médecine égyptienne au temps des pharaons,* 409. The magic value ascribed to this figure may explain why the pagination of the Ebers papyrus runs up to 110 even though it contains only 108 pages.

2. Quotations from: Bontemps, "La médecine en Égypte pharaonique," 23; Balout et al., *La momie de Ramsès II;* Jonckheere, "Le monde des malades dans les textes non médicaux."

3. Masali and Chiarelli, "Demographic Data on the Remains of Ancient Egyptians."

4. Žába, *Les maximes de Ptahhotep,* quoted in Leca, *La médecine égyptienne,* 407.

5. Bontemps, "La médecine en Égypte pharaonique," 152. Leca, *Les Momies.*

6. Herodotus 3:12 (Loeb, 2:14–15).

7. Balout et al., *La momie de Ramsès II.*

8. Hippopotamus fat was a notable ingredient in the Egyptian pharmaco-poeia, mentioned in eight places in Ebers, three places each in Hearst and Ramesseum, and once in Brooklyn. [The Egyptian word *merhet* was used to refer to both animal fats and vegetable oils, whereas *adj* was reserved exclusively for animal fats. Breasted translates the latter term as "grease." The term *merhet* recurs in the passage cited below from Ebers 459.—Trans.]

9. Gray, "Radiography of Ancient Egyptian Mummies." Bucaille, *Les momies des pharaons et la médecine,* 247.

10. Andersen, "The Eye and Its Diseases in Ancient Egypt." Three different terms are used in the papyri to distinguish various degrees of ocular opacity: *hati* (cloudiness), *keku* (darkness), and *akhekhu* (gloom). The remedy for "weakness of sight" is also prescribed to cure *keku* and harmful "actions that develop in the eyes."

11. Ghalioungui, *Magic and Medical Science in Ancient Egypt,* 133. Lefebvre, *Essai sur la médecine égyptienne de l'époque pharaonique,* 83. [Bardinet translates the phrase rendered here as "rise of water" as "a rising up of secretions in the eyes." The condition was treated by ointments and spells: see Ebers 378–380, 385.—Trans.]

12. This bust is now in the Staatliche Museen zu Berlin (no. 21300); see Leca, *La médecine égyptienne,* 295. [It is much more probable that the eye was lost or unfinished, especially in view of the many portraits of Nefertiti that give no indication of cataracts or missing eyes.—Trans.]

13. Riad, *La médecine au temps des pharaons,* 261.

14. See Ghalioungui, "Four Landmarks of Egyptian Cardiology."

15. It has long been supposed that the words *haty* and *ib* are used inter-changeably in the medical papyri to refer to the heart. But Bardinet has established that they refer to distinct concepts. The term *haty* (deriving from a root signifying "before" or "under the command of") refers to the anatomical heart, or cardiac pump, that is responsible for the flow of blood through the human body. The term *ib* has two separate senses. On the one hand it is used in the medical papyri to refer in a general way to the inside of the body and, in this sense, includes all of the internal structures responsible for the vital functions of the organism with the notable exception of the heart *(haty)*. These structures are therefore contained mainly in the thorax and abdomen (jointly designated by the term *shet*). The stomach, regarded as the entrance to this region of the body, is identified by the name *ro-ib*. In the nonmedical papyri, however, *ib* signifies the heart in its spiritual connotation as the seat of thought, memory, and intelligence. It is this organ that stores the memory of actions in life, both good and bad, and that is weighed after death in the ceremony of judgment that takes

place before the tribunal of Osiris. See Bardinet, *Les papyrus médicaux de l'Égypte pharaonique,* 68–81.

16. Ebers 227 mentions a remedy for "driving out the forgetfulness of the heart [the loss of memory], the flight of the heart, and the stinging of the heart," which might correspond either to palpitations or to precordialgia, indeed symptomatic extrasystoles. These are manifested in general by disagreeable pinching sensations in the thorax, by hemithoracic shooting pains that are very localized on the left side, or by the apparent interruption of cardiac rhythm, followed by one or two stronger beats.

17. Other effects of cardiac disorders mentioned include thoracic constriction, where "the heart *(ib)* of the man is choked" (Ebers 855k).

18. Willerson and Teaff, "Egyptian Contributions to Cardiovascular Medicine."

19. Menard, "Les techniques chirurgicales dans l'antiquité égyptienne." Leca, *La médecine égyptienne,* 486. (On the term *sa hemem* see Chapter 1, note 19.)

20. Salem and Eknoyan, "The Kidney in Ancient Egyptian Medicine." Ghanem, "The Urology of Pharaonic Egypt." Nunn, *Ancient Egyptian Medicine,* 92. Like kidney stones, stones formed or retained in the bladder seem to have been uncommon. Of some 30,000 mummies examined by Smith and Dawson, only three instances of renal calculus and two of vesical calculus were found. Ruffer did find three urinary stones in a mummy in which the peripheral presence of phosphates and uric acid could be detected.

21. See Boller and Forbes, "History of Dementia and Dementia in History."

22. Alamovitch and Danziger, *Neurologie,* 88. [The section of Ebers that Bardinet calls the Book of the *Wekhedu* deals with the passage of pathogenic substances through the vessels of the body. Nunn gives it a different name, following the first line of 856a: "Beginning of the 'Book of the Wanderings' *(hebheb)* of *wekhedu* in all the limbs of man . . ." See Nunn, *Ancient Egyptian Medicine,* 61–62.—Trans.]

23. Desroches-Noblecourt, *La femme au temps des pharaons,* 464. Diodorus Siculus 1.80. Andreu, *Images de la vie quotidienne en Égypte au temps des pharaons,* 18–23.

24. Saint-Hilaire, "Note sur un monstre humain trouvé dans les ruines de Thèbes." Smith and Dawson, *Egyptian Mummies.*

25. Dasen, *Dwarfs in Ancient Egypt and Greece,* 126–130. [Another statue showing Seneb with his wife and children, also in the Louvre (JE.51281), is reproduced in Nunn, *Ancient Egyptian Medicine,* 79.—Trans.]

26. Nunn, *Ancient Egyptian Medicine,* 77. Bontemps, "La médecine en Égypte pharaonique," 165. Mention should also be made of a mummy dating from 3700 B.C. discovered at Dashur by Sir Flinders Petrie at the beginning of the twentieth century, whose left femur was narrower than the right femur and shorter by eight centimeters.

27. Desroches-Noblecourt, *Hatchepsout,* 217.

28. Leavesley, "Akhenaten." Weigall, "The Mummy of Akhenaten." [In the case of the statue apparently showing the naked king, it has been argued that this may be a depiction of Akhenaten's wife, Nefertiti. Moreover, we do not know whether Akhenaten actually had any sons, or whether his co-regent was in fact his brother. One theory suggests that Nefertiti was the co-regent under a different throne name. See Montserrat, *Akhenaten,* 48; Malek, *Egypt,* 174.—Trans.]

29. Risse, "Pharaoh Akhenaten of Ancient Egypt."

30. Rinelli, "Diagnostic exacte de la dysmorphie du Pharaon Amenophis IV dit Akhenaton," 72.

31. Derry, "A Case of Hydrocephalus in an Egyptian of the Roman Period." Wreszinski, *Der Papyrus Ebers,* 228.

32. Smith and Dawson, *Egyptian Mummies.* This mummy was mistaken at first for Queen Tiye. Bone analysis yielded an age at death of about twenty-five years, persuading most experts that it was the mummy of Smenkhkara instead.

33. Brothwell and Sandison, *Diseases in Antiquity.* Gray, "Radiography of Ancient Egyptian Mummies." Leca, *La médecine égyptienne,* 322.

34. Wolf, "A Historical Note on the Mode of Administration of Vitamin A for the Cure of Night Blindness." Nunn points out that roasting liver would have reduced its vitamin A content. Ebbell identifies *sharu* as nyctalopia, or night blindness, but Nunn, noting that the hieroglyphic sign for *sharu* does not contain the ideogram for "night," agrees with Ghalioungui that no interpretation more precise than "eye disease" can be sustained. See Nunn, *Ancient Egyptian Medicine,* 200. [Though Nunn was unable to consult Bardinet's translation of the corpus, which appeared when his book was already in press, he was able to check, in addition to the *Grundriss,* a private copy of Ghalioungui's unpublished 1987 translation, which would be the standard version in English today if it were available. Bardinet did not have the opportunity to refer to Ghalioungui's work.—Trans.]

8. Fishermen and Farmers

1. On conditions of daily life generally see Strouhal, *Life in Ancient Egypt,* and Ray, *Reflections of Osiris.*

2. Lalouette, *Au royaume d'Égypte,* 207.

3. Rachet, *Dictionnaire de la civilisation égyptienne,* 200. Andreu, *Images de la vie quotidienne en Égypte au temps des pharaons,* 172.

4. Rachet, *Dictionnaire,* 72. *Satire of the Trades* quoted in Pretre Guignard, "Conditions de travail dans l'Égypte ancienne vues sous l'angle de la médecine du travail," 15. [Also known as the *Instructions of Khety,* the

Satire unfavorably compares with the work of scribes that of masons, goldsmiths, coppersmiths, carpenters, jewelers, stonecutters, potters, bricklayers, builders, vintners, field hands, weavers, reed-cutters, arrow-makers, messengers, furnace-tenders, sandalmakers, barbers, washermen, fowlers, fishermen, and tenant farmers. Even allowing for a considerable degree of bias and exaggeration on the part of the author, it is generally thought to give valuable insight into actual working conditions in ancient Egypt. See Simpson, "Instructions of Khety."—Trans.]

5. Herodotus 2.70 (Sélincourt, 111).

6. This paragraph is also found in Hearst 239 and 241.

7. See the 1993 report of the World Health Organization, cited by Nunn, *Ancient Egyptian Medicine,* 68. The existence of this condition in ancient Egypt was established for the first time by Ruffer in 1910 on the basis of an autopsy of two mummies of the 20th Dynasty.

8. Leca, *La médecine égyptienne au temps des pharaons,* 217.

9. See the discussion of hematuria in Nunn, *Ancient Egyptian Medicine,* 91–92. Bardinet, *Les papyrus médicaux de l'Égypte pharaonique,* 57. In earlier translations of the medical papyri, made during the first half of the twentieth century, the words *wesesh* and *wekha* were mistakenly supposed to refer to "bloody urine." There is general agreement now that they refer to the evacuation or voiding of waste products, with no distinction being made between defecation and micturition.

10. Bardinet has argued that the interpretation of hematuria was not essentially medical, being associated instead with the god Seth. See *Les papyrus médicaux,* 57–58.

11. Brugsch, "Mémoire sur la médecine de l'ancienne Égypte." The *aaa* disease is mentioned 28 times in the Ebers papyrus, 12 times in Berlin, 9 times in Hearst, and once in London. Ebbell and Jonckheere both identified it as urinary schistosomiasis. The fact that the term *aaa* has no connection with any urinary pathology in the nonmedical papyri has forced Egyptologists to revise their opinions, however. See Bardinet, *Les papyrus médicaux,* 135; also Ghalioungui, *La médecine des pharaons,* 74.

12. Jonckheere, *Les médecins de l'Égypte pharaonique.*

13. See Rachet, *Dictionnaire,* 56: "Under the Old Kingdom, all of the land of Egypt was the property of the king and its inhabitants owed the palace taxes, payable in kind or in the form of corvées. Sneferu permanently exempted the cities of his two pyramids from corvées and all other taxes due the king on the condition that his divine cult be perpetuated. Rights and duties were inscribed on a charter [*ar*] and deposited in the royal archives. Such charters were initially granted to the priests responsible for the king's funerary cult and then, from the 5th Dynasty under Neferirkara, to the

temples of the gods. In this way a clergy came into existence that was increasingly independent of the central authorities. Toward the end of the 6th Dynasty similar exemptions were granted to the domains of the provincial governors. These officials founded new cities and granted them charters of immunity, with the result that peasants who had been slaves [*mertu*] gradually became free farmers [*saru*]."

14. Ibid., 200.
15. Quoted in Andreu, *Images de la vie quotidienne*, 149.
16. Leca, *La médecine égyptienne*, 115.
17. Quoted in Andreu, *Images de la vie quotidienne*, 149.
18. Bontemps, "La médecine en Égypte pharaonique," 51.
19. Miller et al., "Diagnosis of *Plasmodium falciparum* Infections in Mummies." Some authors, notably Breasted, had maintained that malaria was not widespread during this period: see Riad, *La médecine au temps des pharaons*, 240.
20. Herodotus 2.95 (Sélincourt, 118).
21. The odorless, yellowish, sweet oil of the moringa tree (*Moringa aptera*) was widely used in Egyptian medicine.—Trans.
22. Ebers 845, 346, 424–429. See also Bardinet, *Les papyrus médicaux*, 313.
23. Ruffer, *Studies in the Paleopathology of Egypt*. Panagiotakopulu, "Pharaonic Egypt and the Origins of Plague."
24. Quoted in Bontemps, "La médecine en Égypte pharaonique."
25. Quoted in ibid.
26. Drioton, "Une représentation de la famine sur un bas relief égyptien de la Ve dynastie." Gray, "Radiography of Ancient Egyptian Mummies."
27. Lefebvre, *Essai sur la médecine égyptienne de l'époque pharaonique*. Hulse, "Leprosy and Ancient Egypt." Browne, "How Old Is Leprosy?" Smith and Derry, "Anatomical Report." Brothwell and Sandison, *Diseases in Antiquity*. Dzierzykray-Rogalski, "Paleopathology of the Ptolemaic Inhabitants of Dakleh Oasis (Egypt)."
28. Tapp, "The Unwrapping of 1770."
29. Horne and Redford, "Aspergillosis and Dracunculosis in Mummies from the Tomb of Parennefer."
30. See, for example, Nunn, *Ancient Egyptian Medicine*, 71.

9. Construction Workers, Miners, Soldiers

1. Slave labor occupied a secondary place in the Egyptian economy, and only developed in Egypt during the New Kingdom following royal campaigns in Nubia and Asia. See Rachet, *Dictionnaire de la civilisation égyptienne*, 103–104, 235.

2. Quoted in Grandet, "La communauté d'artisans de Deir el-Medineh sous les Ramsès."

3. Journal quoted in Della Monica, *La classe ouvrière sous les pharaons*, 125. Archaeological research in the village of Deir el-Medina has yielded valuable information about the life of construction workers; see Černý and Gardiner, *Hieratic Ostraca*.

4. Černý, "A Community of Workmen at Thebes in the Ramessid Period." Boulu, "Le médecin dans la civilisation de l'Égypte pharaonique," 102.

5. Dollfus, "L'ophtalmologie dans l'ancienne Égypte."

6. Jonckheere, "Considération sur l'auxillaire médical pharaonique." Janssen, "Absence from Work by the Necropolis Workmen of Thebes."

7. Breasted, *Edwin Smith Surgical Papyrus*, 1:6. [Breasted notes that the physician's examination of the patient "is conceived as spoken by someone addressing a second person, who is regularly designated by a pronoun in the second person singular. The form of the examination therefore is that of a teacher instructing a pupil that he shall do so and so. This fact raises the question whether this medical roll is not simply an instruction book. The indications are that the treatise has grown up as the product of an effort to record the instructions of the master in the very words he used in the process of instruction." Ibid., 1:38.—Trans.]

8. Edwin Smith 2, 3, 10, 15, 18, 19, 26.

9. Bardinet translates the Egyptian term *wenekh* as "*désajustement,*" which he interprets in case 25 as meaning a complete or partial dislocation: see *Les papyrus médicaux de l'Égypte pharaonique,* 507.—Trans.

10. Andersen, "The Eye and Its Diseases in Ancient Egypt." Ebers 336, 337, 349, 381, 416, 417.

11. Andersen, "The Eye and Its Diseases." Walle and Meulenaere, "Compléments à la prosographie médicale."

12. Mazzone, Banchero, and Esposito, "Neurological Sciences at Their Origin." [Breasted translates *bekenu* as "urine" and notes that the "application of the word 'chest' to the dome of the skull is exactly parallel to the German 'Gehirnkasten'; our own designation 'chest' for the region under the thorax is a similar example of the use of the word to indicate a capacious container and protector of organs." See *Edwin Smith Surgical Papyrus,* 1:197.—Trans.]

13. Nunn, in *Ancient Egyptian Medicine,* 82, interprets the device otherwise, as a wooden chisel not unlike "the boxwood wedge which is still occasionally used to open the mouth in spasm of the jaw," but the instruction to prepare the patient a drink made from earth almonds argues in favor of a feeding tube of the sort proposed by Bardinet in *Les papyrus médicaux,* 499.

14. Thorwald, *Histoire de la médecine dans l'antiquité*, 88. A radiographic study of eighty-eight mummies by P. H. Gray found evidence of bony outgrowth in 57 percent of the cases: see Gray, "Radiography of Ancient Egyptian Mummies." Bontemps, "La médecine en Égypte pharaonique," 182.

15. Della Monica, *La classe ouvrière sous les pharaons*, 125. Stele quoted in Leca, *La médecine égyptienne au temps des pharaons*, 358.

16. Shampo and Kyle, "Medical Mythology."

17. Rachet, *Dictionnaire*, 168. Inscription quoted in Martinez, *Égypte*, 128.

18. Diodorus Siculus 3.12.

19. Gardiner, Peet, and Černý, *The Inscriptions of Sinai*.

20. Anthes, *Die Felseninschriften von Hatnub*, 33–35.

21. Quoted in Gardiner, Peet, and Černý, *Inscriptions of Sinai*.

22. Quoted in Leca, *La médecine égyptienne*.

23. This snake—also known as Aapep or Apophis—is the same snake that according to the *Book of the Dead* attacked Ra.—Trans.

24. Any beneficial effects produced by this remedy would have been psychological rather than physiological: see Nunn, *Ancient Egyptian Medicine*, 189.

25. Leca, *La médecine égyptienne*.

26. Géraut, *L'essentiel des pathologies professionnelles*.

27. Ruffer, *Studies in the Paleopathology of Egypt*. Curry, Anfield, and Tapp, "Electron Microscopy of the Manchester Mummies." Spaeth, "Pneumologie et cancérologie dans la médecine de l'Égypte," 221. Bontemps, "La médecine," 125.

28. This ostracon is catalogued as no. 1091 at the Egyptian Museum in Cairo.

29. Morse, Brothwell, and Ucko, "Tuberculosis in Ancient Egypt." Nesparehan's case involved the destruction of the last four thoracic vertebrae and the first lumbar vertebra, associated with a large abscess extending under the muscle sheath; Ruffer, *Studies in the Paleopathology of Egypt*.

30. Martinez, *Égypte*, 128. Certain texts state that a child ought to have reached a height of two cubits (roughly a meter) before joining the army.

31. Quoted in Erman, *La civilisation égyptienne*, 736. [Erman's English translator, the Oxford Egyptologist Aylward M. Blackman, identifies this text not as a poem but as part of a set of exhortations and warnings to schoolboys from the 19th Dynasty (Anastasi IV.9.4) that, like the *Satire of the Trades*, denigrates soldiering and other professions by comparison with that of the scribe: see Erman, *Literature of the Ancient Egyptians*, 194. Another French version may be found in Lalouette, *Textes sacrés et textes profanes de l'ancienne Égypte*.—Trans.]

32. Diodorus Siculus 1.82 (quoted in Chapter 1).

33. Jonckheere, *Les médecins de l'Égypte pharaonique*. Bardinet, *Les papyrus médicaux*, 258.

34. Erman, *La civilisation égyptienne*, 702. On the *hemem* and related surgical instruments see Nunn, *Ancient Egyptian Medicine*, 164–167.

35. Hauben and Sonneveld, "The Influence of War on the Development of Plastic Surgery"; see also Sanchez, "Injuries in the Battle of Kadesh" and "A Neurosurgeon's View of the Battle Reliefs of King Sety I." Quotation from Lefebvre, *Essai sur la médecine égyptienne de l'époque pharaonique*. Edwin Smith 44 describes a fracture of several ribs associated with a chest wound that may have been caused by a sharp object with a broad edge such as an axe or a double-edged sword. The prognosis of this injury is grave ("An ailment for which nothing can be done") in view of attendant pneumothorax and subcutaneous emphysema (accumulation of air in the chest cavity and the tissues beneath the skin).

36. Risse, "Rational Egyptian Surgery." Knoeller and Seifried, "Historical Perspective."

37. See also Edwin Smith 4, 5, 7.

38. Sullivan, "The Identity and Work of the Ancient Egyptian Surgeon." Edwin Smith 4 reports a case of otorrhea ("[one] who loses blood from the nostrils and the ears"), undoubtedly due to a fracture of the otic bone, the prognosis of which is always very pessimistic. The practitioner is therefore required to abstain from all therapeutic intervention, limiting himself to monitoring the development of the traumatism, while keeping the patient in a seated position with the aid of brick supports.

39. Ghalioungui, *Magic and Medical Science in Ancient Egypt*, 92–93. Batrawi, "The Pyramid Studies." Menard, "Les techniques chirurgicales dans l'antiquité égyptienne." Pahl, "La tomographie par ordinateur appliquée aux momies égyptiennes."

40. Menard, "Les techniques chirurgicales," 63.

41. Leca, *La médecine égyptienne*, 433–434. On the structure of the circulatory system constituted by the heart *(haty)* and vessels *(metu)* see Bardinet, *Les papyrus médicaux*, 117–119.

42. Bardinet interprets the phrase "moor him at his mooring post" to mean simply that the patient was confined to bed. Breasted's more expansive commentary draws a stronger conclusion: "In the latter part of the Old Kingdom, probably not later than 2500 B.C., some 'modern' surgeon, as unknown to us as the original author, equipped the document with a commentary in the form of brief definitions and explanations, which we term glosses, appended to each case. For example, when the original treatise directed the practitioner to 'moor [the patient] at his mooring stakes,' the commentator knows that this curious idiom is no longer intelligible and

appends the explanation, 'It means put him on his accustomed diet and do not administer to him any medicine.'" Breasted, *Edwin Smith Surgical Papyrus,* 1:10.—Trans.

43. Vikentieff, "Deux rites du jubilé royal à l'époque protodynastique."

44. Diodorus Siculus 1.78 (Loeb, 1:268–269). Leca, *La médecine égyptienne,* 434.

45. Brothwell and Møller-Christensen, "A Possible Case of Amputation Dated c. 2000 B.C.," cited in Leca, *La médecine égyptienne,* 434. Gray, "Radiography of Ancient Egyptian Mummies."

46. Bellouard, "Le dossier médical des pharaons de la Haute Époque," 45.

47. On this forensic analysis as evidence of a major battle against the Hyksos during Seqenenra's reign, see Bourriau, "The Second Intermediate Period," 211. Manfred Bietak and Eugen Strouhal argued that the wounds were caused by bronze weapons similar to those used by the Hyksos, against whom Seqenenra went to war after their king, Apophis, called the pharaoh and his two sons the "bellowing hippopotamuses of Luxor." See "Die Todesumstände des Pharaohs Seqenenre (siebzehnte Dynastie)."

48. Bellouard, "Le dossier médical," 45. Bietak and Strouhal, while agreeing that Seqenenra's injuries were not inflicted simultaneously, hold that the angles of the wounds argue for death in combat, the pharaoh having been forced to his knees.

49. Bucaille, *Les momies des pharaons et la médecine,* 247. Shattock, "Minutes of a Meeting of the Pathological Section of the Royal Society of Medicine." Bellouard, "Le dossier médical," 71. [The Exodus, usually thought to have taken place between 1250 and 1200 B.C., is unmentioned in Egyptian documents. The so-called Israel Stele, discovered in Merenptah's funerary temple in 1896, refers to Israel as an already established society in Palestine by year 5 of his reign, which has led many scholars to place the Exodus during the reign of Rameses II. See David and David, *Biographical Dictionary of Ancient Egypt,* 78.—Trans.]

10. Bakers, Priests, Scribes, Embalmers, Prostitutes

1. Menard, "Les techniques chirurgicales dans l'antiquité égyptienne," 111. Samuel, "Cereal Foods and Nutrition in Ancient Egypt."

2. Erman, *La civilisation égyptienne,* 255. Pretre Guignard, "Conditions de travail dans l'Égypte ancienne vues sous l'angle de la médecine du travail," 16. Géraut, *L'essentiel des pathologies professionnelles,* 54.

3. Ebbell, *The Papyrus Ebers,* 67–68.

4. Scarborough, "On Medications for Burns in Classical Antiquity." Shampo and Kyle, "Medical Mythology."

5. Nickol et al., "An Examination of the Dental State of an Egyptian

Mummy by Means of Computer Tomography." Leek, "Teeth and Bread in Ancient Egypt." Schwartz, "La médecine dentaire dans l'Égypte pharaonique." Marion, "Dentistry of Ancient Egypt."

6. Pierre-François Puech has argued that "the marked erosion of the teeth is chiefly due to the nutrients and silica found in plants rather than the result of specks of dust and grains of sand [and other impurities in] the food." Puech, "Autopsie d'une momie égyptienne," 47.

7. Thus, at the end of the 20th Dynasty, the high priest of Amun, Herihor, was successively vizier and chief general of the army, and on the death of Rameses XI went so far as to assume royal titles. By the Late Period the priesthood was the largest landholder in Egypt; see Rachet, *Dictionnaire de la civilisation égyptienne*, 61–62.

8. Ibid., 215.

9. Martinez, *Égypte*, 124. Morenz, *La religion égyptienne*. Erman, *La civilisation égyptienne*, 382.

10. Amherst papyrus quoted in Peet, *The Great Tomb Robberies of the Twentieth Egyptian Dynasty*, 103. Boulu, "Le médecin dans la civilisation de l'Égypte pharaonique," 106. Herodotus 2.37 (Sélincourt, 99–100).

11. Sauneron, *Les prêtres de l'ancienne Égypte*.

12. See Darby, Ghalioungui, and Grivetti, *Food*.

13. Zimmerman, "The Paleopathology of the Cardiovascular System." Thorwald, *Histoire de la médecine dans l'antiquité*, 43. Balout et al., *La momie de Ramsès II*. A study by Ruffer of mummies (or fragments of mummies) of twenty-one priests and priestesses of Amun from the 21st Dynasty, found at Deir el-Bahri, revealed six cases of atherosclerosis. A later study, carried out in 1975 by a team led by Aidan Cockburn on the mummy of a priest from the Ptolemaic Period (PUM II) who died at the age of 35–40 in 170 A.D., disclosed diffuse atheromatous aortic plaques as well as a thickening of the intima in the narrowest arteries typical of an atheromatous condition. See Cockburn et al., "Autopsy of an Egyptian Mummy."

14. Examination of the mummy of Nesptah, barber of Amun, a low-level functionary in the temple of Amun at Karnak (now in the Boston Museum of Fine Arts), revealed extensive distal calcifications in the internal iliac, femoral, and anterior and posterior tibial arteries. See Marx and D'Auria, "CT Examination of Eleven Egyptian Mummies."

15. Sarazin, "La pathologie cardio-vasculaire dans l'Égypte ancienne," 90.

16. Spaeth, "Pneumologie et cancérologie dans la médecine de l'Égypte," 223. Balout, "L'opération Ramsès II."

17. On the hardening of vessels in the context of Egyptian physiology see Bardinet, *Les papyrus médicaux de l'Égypte pharaonique*, 67–68.

18. Rachet, *Dictionnaire*, 237.

19. Ibid., 122. [Generally speaking, from the end of the New Kingdom onward, only hieratic was taught to scribes, the writing of hieroglyphs having by this point become the specialized task of an elite and much smaller group.—Trans.]

20. *The Satire of the Trades,* quoted in ibid., 238.

21. Rose, Armelagos, and Perry, "Dental Anthropology of the Nile Valley." Nickol et al., "An Examination of the Dental State of an Egyptian Mummy." Nunn, *Ancient Egyptian Medicine*, 203.

22. El-Mahdy, *Momies, mythes et magie,* 87. Balout et al., *La momie de Ramsès II.* Batrawi, "The Pyramid Studies."

23. Anastasi IV quoted in Etaric, "L'alimentation et ses répercussions sur la sphère bucco-dentaire dans l'Égypte ancienne," 37.

24. Interpreting the use of honey, prescribed in Ebers 740 and 741, is a trickier matter.

25. Thekkaniyil et al., "Dental and Skeletal Findings on an Ancient Egyptian Mummy." Quenouille, "L'art dentaire dans l'Égypte ancienne."

26. Quenouille, "L'art dentaire." Etaric, "L'alimentation et ses répercussions," 62. Weinberger, "The Dental Art in Ancient Egypt." Leek, "Observations on a Collection of Crania from the Mastabas of the Reign of Cheops at Giza."

27. Ruffer, *Studies in the Paleopathology of Egypt.*

28. The incidence of gastroenterological disorders is less certain owing to a common mistranslation of the term *ro-ib*, which has traditionally been identified with the stomach. Paragraphs 189, 198, 199, and 206 in Ebers, in particular, have therefore wrongly been understood as describing gastric disorders. See Bardinet, *Les papyrus médicaux,* 167–172.

29. Smith and Dawson, *Egyptian Mummies.* Gray, "Radiography of Ancient Egyptian Mummies."

30. Banov, "The Chester Beatty Medical Papyrus." Viso and Uriach, "The 'Guardians of the Anus' and Their Practice."

31. The ripe sycamore fig (*Ficus sycomorus*) was "notched" in order to allow parasites (presumably the source of the nausea mentioned earlier in those who ate the uncut fruit) to escape. See Mannliche, *An Ancient Egyptian Herbal,* 103.

32. Revelat, "Pensées et pratiques médicales de l'Égypte pharaonique."

33. See in this connection Banov, "Proctology in Ancient Egypt."

34. Lethor, "Du coeur et des vaisseaux dans l'Égypte ancienne," 59.

35. Diodorus Siculus 1.91 (Loeb, 1:310–311).

36. Herodotus 2.89 (Sélincourt, 116).

37. Moutet, "Fossoyeurs et services funéraires." Géraut, *L'essentiel des pathologies professionnelles,* 182–183.

38. See Bardinet, *Les papyrus médicaux,* 193–197.
39. Ghalioungui, *La médecine des pharaons,* 339.
40. Tapp, "Disease in the Manchester Mummies." Horne and Lewin, "Autopsy of an Egyptian Mummy." Cockburn et al., "Autopsy of an Egyptian Mummy."
41. Lefebvre, *Essai sur la médecine égyptienne de l'époque pharaonique.*
42. See the commentary in Bardinet, *Les papyrus médicaux,* 52–53. [Nunn takes *isw* to refer to a rush- or grass-like plant of the genus *Carex,* found in marshy places. Bardinet translates the word more generally as "reed" and, unlike Nunn, gives no dosage for pyrethrum.—Trans.]
43. No Egyptian term seems clearly to correspond to pinworms, though Leca has argued that Berlin 11 specifies a treatment for this species in the form of an ointment to be applied to the anus. See Leca, *La médecine égyptienne au temps des pharaons,* 213.
44. Andersen, "The Eye and Its Diseases in Ancient Egypt."
45. Herodotus 2.121.
46. Herodotus 2.126 (Sélincourt, 132–133).
47. Quoted in Leca, *La médecine égyptienne,* 423. The Egyptian word for a prostitute was *khenemet:* see Desroches-Noblecourt, *La femme au temps des pharaons,* 372.
48. Cianfrani, *Short History of Obstetrics and Gynecology,* 24–37.
49. Morice, "La gynécologie et l'obstétrique en Égypte pharaonique," 127–128. Bardis, "Contraception in Ancient Egypt."
50. Morice et al., "Gynécologie et obstétrique dans l'ancienne Égypte." Granville, "An Essay on Egyptian Mummies with Observations on the Art of Embalming among the Ancient Egyptians." A mummy found in the necropolis of Dush (no. 64212—plate VIIb) bears traces of a right inguinal incision that suggests suppurative adenitis. It also has a voluminous left vaginal lip that may indicate bartholinitis with secondary adenitis.
51. Leca, *La médecine égyptienne,* 322.

Epilogue: Transmission of Egyptian Medical Knowledge

1. Maspero, *Le papyrus Ebers et la médecine égyptienne,* 287.
2. Homer, *The Odyssey,* 4.229–232, trans. Murray, 1:134–135. [Paeëon (also Paean or Paeon) is the physician of the gods in Greek myth, and an epithet for Asclepius.—Trans.]
3. Herodotus 3.1 (Sélincourt, 154).
4. Herodotus 3.129 (Sélincourt, 204).
5. Herodotus 3.131, 3.130 (Sélincourt, 205, 204).
6. Jonckheere, *Les médecins de l'Égypte pharaonique,* 81. Niqmad quoted in Ghalioungui, *La médecine des pharaons,* 77. Boulu, "Le médecin dans la civilisation de l'Égypte pharaonique," 196.

7. See Gardiner, *The Kadesh Inscriptions of Ramesses II*. Quotation from Kitchen, *Pharaoh Triumphant*, 92.

8. Kitchen, *Pharaoh Triumphant*, 91, 82.

9. Boulu, "Le médecin," 201. [The story of this princess is related by the famous Bentresh stele, discovered by Champollion at Karnak and now in the Louvre. Its inscription, while purporting to date from the reign of Rameses II, was composed sometime between the fourth and second centuries B.C.—Trans.]

10. Contenau, *La médecine en Assyrie et en Babylonie*, 197.

11. Vercoutter, *Essai sur les relations entre Égyptiens et Préhellènes*, 88. Bardinet, "Remarques sur les maladies de la peau." Goedicke cited in Boulu, "Le médecin," 201.

12. Gabriel-Leroux, *Les premières civilisations de la Méditerranée*, 96. Lloyd, "The Late Period," 374–376. Nunn, *Ancient Egyptian Medicine*, 206.

13. Sauneron, *Les prêtres de l'ancienne Égypte*, 111.

14. Quoted in Boulu, "Le médecin." [Even the earliest sources for Plato's visit to Egypt, Cicero and Diodorus, are quite late, casting doubt on the veracity of the tradition. Clement says that Plato was a disciple of Sechnuphis of Heliopolis, just as Pythagoras, who was also said to have traveled to Phoenicia and Babylonia, had been taught by Sonchis, the "highest prophet of the Egyptians" (*Stromateis* 1.15.69.1). It seems likely that the story of instruction in the secrets of the Egyptians was inserted into Plato's biography to show that he was Pythagoras's equal in mastering the wisdom of the East, though detractors pointed to it as proof of Plato's lack of originality. Early Christian writers saw Egypt as the place where Plato acquired knowledge of the Hebrew Old Testament, especially the Book of Moses. See Riginos, *Platonica*, 64–69.—Trans.]

15. Yoyotte, "Une théorie étiologique des médecins égyptiens." [The case for direct influence was made by Robert O. Steuer in "Whdw: Aetiological Principle of Pyaemia in Ancient Egyptian Medicine," and by Steuer and Saunders, in *Ancient Egyptian and Cnidean Medicine*. Their arguments have been forcefully rebutted by Bardinet in *Les papyrus médicaux de l'Égypte pharaonique*, 128–135. See too the more sympathetic discussion in Nunn, *Ancient Egyptian Medicine*, 61–62.—Trans.]

16. Frommeyer, "Commentaries on the History of Medicine." Martiny, *Hippocrate et la médecine*, 63.

17. Carlsberg IV, 2; V, 1; VII, 2; see also Leca, *La médecine égyptienne au temps des pharaons*, 326–327. [In the Hippocratic treatise *Generation/ Nature of the Child* 2, sperm is said to originate in the brain, whence it travels down along the spinal cord.—Trans.]

18. Hippocrates, *On Joints* 58 (Loeb, 3:338–339); *Aphorisms* 6.38 (Loeb, 4:188–189). Edwin Smith 5, 8, 13, 22, 33–44.

19. Hippocrates, *Aphorisms* 1.20 (Loeb, 4:106–107). Edwin Smith 3, 5, 19, 21, 28, 29. On the mooring post see Chapter 9, note 42.
20. Nunn, *Ancient Egyptian Medicine,* 206. Von Staden, *Herophilus,* 29. Yoyotte, "Une théorie étiologique."
21. Remondon, "Problèmes de bilinguisme dans l'Égypte lagide (UPZ, I, 48)." Préaux, "Les prescriptions médicales des ostracas grecs de la bibliothèque Bodléenne."
22. Yahuda, "Medical and Anatomical Terms in the Pentateuch in the Light of Egyptian Medical Papyri."
23. Ibid. Weill, "Les transmissions littéraires d'Égypte à Israël," 43. Georges Posener has found 680 mentions of Egypt in the Bible: see *Dictionnaire de la civilisation égyptienne.*
24. That is, "in the manner of the Egyptians," as the French translation of this verse has it.—Trans.
25. Recall from Chapter 3, however, that Herodotus (2.86) says the process took seventy days.—Trans.
26. Hearst 172; see Bardinet, *Les papyrus médicaux,* 188, 212; and Faulkner, *A Concise Dictionary of Middle Egyptian,* 238.
27. Ghalioungui, *La médecine des pharaons.*

Primary Sources for Egyptian Medicine

1. *Théma: Encyclopédie Larousse,* vol. 1, 37. An estimate of 400,000 volumes at the end of the reign of Ptolemy II Philadelphus is given by Lerman in "L'école de médecine d'Alexandrie," 32.
2. Spaeth, "Pneumologie et cancérologie dans la médecine de l'Égypte." [The evolution of Egyptian, a branch of the Afro-Asiatic family of languages, is conventionally divided into five periods: Old Egyptian (ca. 3000–2200 B.C.), Middle Egyptian (ca. 2200–1600 B.C.), Late Egyptian (ca. 1500–700 B.C.), Demotic (ca. 700 B.C.–400 A.D.), and Coptic (ca. 100–1400 A.D.). Three principal systems of writing are distinguished: hieroglyphic, hieratic, and demotic. Hieroglyphic, based on stylized drawings, was reserved mainly for texts engraved or painted on monuments, stelae, and objects, and used from the earliest period of Egyptian culture until the fourth century A.D. Hieratic is a simplified form of the hieroglyphic style. From the beginning of the 21st Dynasty until the Roman Period, when it disappeared, hieratic was used for writing sacred and profane texts on papyri and ostraca. Demotic appeared in the eighth century B.C. as a means for transcribing the demotic tongue. The last known inscription in this style is dated to A.D. 452. Coptic, the culminating phase in the development of the Egyptian language, emerged with the Christianization of

Egypt in the first century A.D. and, in its written form, used a modified Greek alphabet. It survives today as the liturgical language of the Christian Coptic community.—Trans.]

3. Ibid., 43. On Champollion's achievement see Iversen, *The Myth of Egypt and Its Hieroglyphics in European Tradition*, 133–145.

4. Bardinet, "Les papyrus de l'Égypte ancienne." For an overview of the history and interpretation of the medical papyri see the introduction to Bardinet's volume of translation and commentary, *Les papyrus médicaux de l'Égypte pharaonique*, 13–29.

5. Leca, *La médecine égyptienne au temps des pharaons*, 21. Ebers, *Papyros Ebers*.

6. See Bardinet, *Les papyrus médicaux*, 81–113; also Nunn, *Ancient Egyptian Medicine*, 45–49. Thorwald, *Histoire de la médecine dans l'antiquité*, 49.

7. Nunn, *Ancient Egyptian Medicine*, 25.

8. Breasted, *The Edwin Smith Surgical Papyrus*. [Nunn notes that the tomb from which the Ebers papyrus was taken, thought to have been in the Assassif area of the Theban necropolis on the west bank of the Nile across from Luxor, has never actually been identified. "It can only be speculated," he emphasizes, "that it came from the tomb of a doctor, and it is possible that it may have come from the same tomb as the Edwin Smith" (*Ancient Egyptian Medicine*, 30).—Trans.]

9. Reisner, *The Hearst Medical Papyrus*. Wreszinski, *Der Londoner medizinische Papyrus (Brit. Museum nr. 10,059) und der Papyrus Hearst in Transkription*.

10. Wreszinski, *Der grosse medizinische Papyrus des Berliner Museums*. Quotation in Leca, *La médecine égyptienne*, 31.

11. Leca, *La médecine égyptienne*.

12. Griffith, *The Petrie Papyri;* see also Stevens, "Gynaecology from Ancient Egypt." Von den Driesch, "Is There a Veterinary Papyrus of Kahun?"

13. Wreszinski, *Der Londoner medizinische Papyrus*.

14. An English translation by Gardiner can be found in *Hieratic Papyri in the British Museum*, 3rd series, nos. 53–54.

15. Massart, *The Leiden Magical Papyrus I 343 and I 345*.

16. Griffith and Thompson, *The Demotic Magical Papyrus of London and Leiden*.

17. Sauneron, *Un traité égyptien d'ophiologie*.

18. Iversen, *Papyrus Carlsberg No. VIII*. Ray, "Papyrus Carlsberg 67."

19. Gardiner, *The Ramesseum Papyri*.

20. Newberry, *The Amherst Papyri;* the medical papyrus is now at the Pierpont Morgan Library in New York. The Anastasi papyrus now in the

British Museum, was first published by Dawson in the *Journal of Egyptian Archeology* in 1944. Lexa, *Papyrus Insinger;* see also Lichtheim, *Late Egyptian Wisdom Literature in the International Context.* Goyon, *Le papyrus du Louvre n° 3279.* Erman, *Die Märchen des Papyrus Westcar.* The Vatican papyrus was first published by Suys in *Orientalia* in 1934. Reymond, *From the Contents of the Libraries of the Suchos Temples in the Fayyum.*

21. Gardiner, *Royal Canon of Turin;* Pleyte and Rossi, *Papyrus de Turin.*
22. Spaeth, "Pneumologie et cancérologie," 55–56.
23. Anthes, *Die Felseninschriften von Hatnub.*
24. Boulu, "Le médecin dans la civilisation de l'Égypte pharaonique," 11.
25. Nunn, *Ancient Egyptian Medicine,* 164–165.
26. Leca, *La médecine égyptienne,* 40–41.

Interpreting the Ten Plagues of Egypt

1. Trémillon, "Essai d'interprétation des plaies d'Égypte," 79.
2. Ibid., 24. Millo, "La mort chez les Égyptiens," 143.
3. Trémillon, "Essai d'interprétation," 31.
4. Fage, *Commentaires sur la première plaie d'Égypte.* Trémillon, "Essai d'interprétation," 32.
5. See Bourdial and Coquart, "L'éruption d'un volcan expliquerait les 10 plaies d'Égypte."
6. Ibid. Trémillon, "Essai d'interprétation," 35.
7. Exodus 8:16–19. The King James Version has "lice," the Revised Standard Version "gnats."—Trans.
8. Leca, *La médecine égyptienne au temps des pharaons.* Gemayel, *L'hygiène et la médecine à travers la Bible.* Balout et al., *La momie de Ramsès II.*
9. Millo, "La mort chez les Égyptiens," 145.
10. Bourdial and Coquart, "L'éruption d'un volcan."
11. Trémillon, "Essai d'interprétation," 49.
12. Ibid., 35. Bourdial and Coquart, "L'éruption d'un volcan."
13. Dols, "Plague in Early Islamic History."
14. Levin, "Death of the First-Born."
15. Bourdial and Coquart, "L'éruption d'un volcan."
16. Wein, "The Plagues of Egypt."
17. Nof and Paldor, "Are There Oceanographic Explanations for the Israelites' Crossing of the Red Sea?" cited in Bourdial and Coquart, "L'éruption d'un volcan."

Works Cited

Ackerknecht, Erwin H. "Paleopathology." In *Anthropology Today: An Encyclopedic Inventory*, ed. A. L. Kroeber, 120–126. Chicago: University of Chicago Press, 1953.

Alamovitch, Sonia, and Nicolas Danziger. *Neurologie*. Paris: Estem-Medline, 1995.

Andersen, S. R. "The Eye and Its Diseases in Ancient Egypt." *Acta Ophthalmologica Scandinavica* 75 (1997): 338–344.

Andreu, Guillemette. *Images de la vie quotidienne en Égypte au temps des pharaons*. Paris: Hachette, 1997.

Anthes, Rudolf. *Die Felseninschriften von Hatnub*. Leipzig: Hinrichs, 1928.

Les artistes de pharaon. Paris: Éditions de la Réunion des Musées Nationaux, 2002.

Assmann, Jan. *Images et rites de la mort dans l'Égypte ancienne*. Paris: Cybèle, 2000.

Atta, H. M. "Edwin Smith Surgical Papyrus: The Oldest Known Surgical Treatise." *American Surgeon* 65 (1999): 1190–1192.

Baldock, C., S. W. Hughes, D. K. Whittaker, J. Taylor, R. Davis, A. J. Spencer, K. Tonge, and A. Sofat. "3-D Reconstruction of an Ancient Egyptian Mummy Using X-Ray Computer Tomography." *Journal of the Royal Society of Medicine* 87 (1994): 806–808.

Balout, L. "L'opération Ramsès II: contribution des laboratoires à l'égyptologie." *Bulletin de la Société française d'égyptologie* 83 (1978): 8–23.

Balout, Lionel, et al., eds. *La momie de Ramsès II: contribution scientifique à l'égyptologie*. Paris: Éditions Recherche sur les civilisations, 1985.

Banov, L., Jr. "The Chester Beatty Medical Papyrus: The Earliest Known Treatise Completely Devoted to Anorectal Disease." *Surgery* 58 (1965): 1037–1043.

———. "Proctology in Ancient Egypt: Its Continuing Influence on the Management of Anorectal Disease." *Southern Medical Journal* 58 (1965): 1366–1369.

Bardinet, Thierry. *Dents et mâchoires dans les représentations religieuses et la pratique médicale de l'Égypte ancienne.* Rome: Pontificio Istituto Biblico, 1990.

———. "Le mot *bââ*, dans les papyrus médicaux de l'Égypte pharaonique." In *Leçons d'histoire de la médecine,* ed. Danielle Gourevitch. Paris: Ellipses, 1995.

———. "Les médecins dans la société égyptienne à l'époque des pharaons: mythe et réalité." *Medecina nei secoli* 9 (1997): 177–188.

———. "Les papyrus de l'Égypte ancienne." *Pour la science* 226 (1996): 60–66.

———. *Les papyrus médicaux de l'Égypte pharaonique: traduction intégrale et commentaire.* Paris: Fayard, 1995.

———. "Remarques sur les maladies de la peau, la lèpre et le châtiment dans l'Égypte ancienne." *Revue d'égyptologie* 39 (1988): 3–36.

Bardis, P. "Contraception in Ancient Egypt." *Centaurus* 12 (1968): 305–307.

Barns, John W. B., ed. *Five Ramesseum Papyri.* Oxford: Printed for the Griffith Institute at the University Press, 1956.

Barraco, Robin A. "Paleobiochemistry." In *Mummies, Disease, and Ancient Cultures,* rev. 2nd ed., ed. Aidan Cockburn, Eve Cockburn, and Theodore A. Reyman (Cambridge: Cambridge University Press, 1998), 312–326.

Barraco, R. A., T. A. Reyman, and A. Cockburn, "Paleobiochemical Analysis of an Egyptian Mummy." *Journal of Human Evolution* 6 (1977): 533–546.

Baslez, Louis. "Les poisons dans l'antiquité égyptienne." Doctoral thesis in medicine, University of Paris, 1932.

Batrawi, A. "The Pyramid Studies: Anatomical Reports." *Annales du service des antiquités de l'Égypte* 47 (1947): 97–111.

Bellouard, Arnauld. "Le dossier médical des pharaons de la Haute Époque." Doctoral thesis in medicine, University of Paris VI-Broussais, 1986.

Belmondo, Paul. "Nosologie égyptienne." Doctoral thesis in medicine, University of Aix-Marseille, 1989.

Bietak, Manfred, and Eugen Strouhal. "Die Todesumstände des Pharaohs Seqenenre (siebzehnte Dynastie)." *Annalen des Naturhistorischen Museum Wien* 78 (1974): 29–52.

Birkett, D. A., C. L. Gummer, and R. P. R. Dawber. "Preservation of the Sub-Cellular Ultrastructure of Ancient Hair." In David, ed., *Science in Egyptology,* 367–369.

Bloomfield, J. A. "Radiology of Egyptian Mummy." *Australasian Radiology Journal* 29 (1985): 64–66.

Boller, F., and M. M. Forbes. "History of Dementia and Dementia in History: An Overview." *Journal of the Neurological Sciences* 58 (1998): 125–133.

Bontemps, Gonzague. "La médecine en Égypte pharaonique." Doctoral thesis in medicine, University of Angers, 1990.

Boulu, Gilles. "Le médecin dans la civilisation de l'Égypte pharaonique." Doctoral thesis in medicine, University of Amiens, 1990.

Bourdial, L., and J. Coquart. "L'éruption d'un volcan expliquerait les 10 plaies d'Égypte." *Science et vie* 1016 (2002): 46–61.

Bourriau, Janine. "The Second Intermediate Period." In Shaw, ed., *Oxford History of Ancient Egypt,* 185–217.

Bowman, W. C. "Drugs Ancient and Modern." *Scottish Medical Journal* 24 (1979): 131–140.

Boyd, W. C. "Les groupes sanguins chez les anciens égyptiens." *Chronique d'Égypte* 23 (1937): 41–44.

Breasted, James Henry, ed. *The Edwin Smith Surgical Papyrus, Published in Facsimile and Hieroglyphic Transliteration with Translation and Commentary in Two Volumes.* Chicago: University of Chicago Press, 1930.

Brier, B., and R. Wade. "The Use of Natron in Egyptian Mummification: Preliminary Report." *Paleopathology Newsletter* 89 (1995): 7–9.

Brothwell, Don R., and A. T. Sandison, eds. *Diseases in Antiquity: A Survey of the Diseases, Injuries, and Surgery of Early Populations.* Springfield, Ill.: Charles C. Thomas, 1967.

Brothwell, D. R., and V. Møller-Christensen. "A Possible Case of Amputation Dated c. 2000 B.C." *Man* 63 (1963): 192–194.

Browne, S. G. "How Old Is Leprosy?" *International Journal of Dermatology* 19(1980): 530–532.

Brugsch, H. F. K. "Mémoire sur la médecine de l'ancienne Égypte." *Allgemeine Monatsschrift für Wissenschaft und Lit'* (1853): 44–56.

Brunner, Hellmut. "L'éducation en ancienne Égypte." In *Histoire mondiale de l'éducation,* ed. Gaston Mialaret and Jean Vial, 1:65–86. Paris: Presses Universitaires de France, 1987.

Bucaille, Maurice. *Les momies des pharaons et la médecine.* Paris: Séguier, 1987.

Buckley, S. A., A. W. Stott, and R. P. Evershed. "Studies of Organic Residues from Ancient Egyptian Mummies Using High Temperature–Gas Chromotography–Mass Spectrometry." *Analyst* 124 (1999): 443–452.

Caton, R. "The Medicine and the Medicine God of the Egyptians." *Lancet* (25 June 1904): 1769–1772.

Černý, J. "A Community of Workmen at Thebes in the Ramessid Period." *Bulletin de l'Institut français d'archéologie orientale* 50 (1973): 35.

———. "Quelques ostracas hiératiques inédits de Thèbes au musée du Caire." *Annales du service des antiquités de l'Égypte* 27 (1927): 183–210.

Černý, Jaroslav, and Alan H. Gardiner. *Hieratic Ostraca*. Oxford: Griffith Institute, 1957.

Chabas, F. "De la circumcision chez les Égyptiens." *Revue d'archéologie* 3 (1861): 298–300.

Champdor, Albert. *Le livre des morts: papyrus d'Any, de Hunefer, d'Anhaï du British Museum*. Paris: Albin Michel, 1963.

Chapel, T. A., A. H. Mehregan, and T. A. Reyman. "Histologic Findings in Mummified Skin." *Journal of the American Academy of Dermatology* 4 (1981): 27–30.

Cianfrani, Theodore. *A Short History of Obstetrics and Gynecology*. Springfield, Ill.: Charles C. Thomas, 1960.

Clement of Alexandria. *Stromateis*. Books 1–3. Trans. John Ferguson. Washington: Catholic University of America Press, 1991.

Cockburn, A., R. A. Barraco, T. A. Reyman, and W. H. Peck. "Autopsy of an Egyptian Mummy." *Science* 187 (1975): 1155–1160.

Connolly, R. C. "Kinship of Smenkhkare and Tutankhamon Demonstrated Serologically." *Nature* 224 (1969): 325–326.

Contenau, Georges. *La médecine en Assyrie et en Babylonie*. Paris: Maloine, 1938.

Curry, A., C. Anfield, and E. Tapp. "Electron Microscopy of the Manchester Mummies." In David, ed., *Manchester Museum Mummy Project*, 103–111.

Darby, William J., Paul Ghalioungui, and Louis Grivetti. *Food: The Gift of Osiris*. 2 vols. London: Academic Press, 1977.

Dasen, Véronique. *Dwarfs in Ancient Egypt and Greece*. Oxford: Clarendon Press, 1993.

Daumas, François. *La civilisation de l'Égypte pharaonique*. Paris: Arthaud, 1987.

———. "Le sanatorium de Dendera." *Bulletin de l'Institut français d'archéologie orientale* 56 (1957): 35–37.

David, Ann Rosalie, ed. "Disease in Egyptian Mummies: The Contribution of New Technologies." *Lancet* 349 (1997): 1760–1763.

———, ed. *The Manchester Museum Mummy Project*. Manchester: University of Manchester Press, 1979.

———. "Mummification." In Nicholson and Shaw, eds., *Ancient Egyptian Materials and Technology*, 372–389.

———. "Mummification." In Redford, ed., *The Ancient Gods Speak*, 231–237.

———, ed. *Science in Egyptology*. Manchester: Manchester University Press, 1986.

David, Rosalie, and Antony E. David. *Biographical Dictionary of Ancient Egypt*. London: Seaby, 1992.

Davies, W. Vivian, and Roxie Walker, eds. *Biological Anthropology and the Study of Ancient Egypt*. London: British Museum Press, 1993.

Dawson, W. R. "The Anastasi Papyrus." *Journal of Egyptian Archeology* 35 (1944): 158–166.

De Bidart, Hélène. "Momification et paléopathologie des momies de l'Égypte ancienne." Doctoral thesis in medicine, University of Nancy I, 1998.

Della Monica, Madeleine. *La classe ouvrière sous les pharaons*. Paris: Maisonneuve, 1975.

Derry, D. E. "A Case of Hydrocephalus in an Egyptian of the Roman Period." *Journal of Anatomy and Physiology* 47 (1912–1913): 436–458.

Desroches-Noblecourt, Christiane. *Hatchepsout*. Paris: Pygmalion, 2002.

———. *La femme au temps des pharaons*. Paris: Stock/L. Pernoud, 1986.

Diodorus Siculus. *The Library of History*. Trans. C. H. Oldfather. Loeb Classical Library, 12 vols. Cambridge, Mass.: Harvard University Press, 1933–1967.

Dioscorides. *The Greek Herbal of Dioscorides*. Trans. John Goodyer, ed. R. T. Gunther. New York: Hafner, 1959.

Dollfus, M.-A. "Les connaissances neurologiques des anciens égyptiens." *Presse médicale* 19 (1939): 2.

———. "L'ophtalmologie dans l'ancienne Égypte." *Bulletin de la société française d'égyptologie* 49 (1967): 12–23.

Dols, M. W. "Plague in Early Islamic History." *Journal of the Oriental Society* 3 (1974): 371–384.

Driesch, A. von den. "Is There a Veterinary Papyrus of Kahun?" *Historia Medicinae Veterineriae* 26 (2001): 105–106.

Drioton, E. "Une représentation de la famine sur un bas relief égyptien de la Ve dynastie." *Bulletin de l'Institut d'Égypte* 25 (1942): 44–45.

Dunand, Françoise, and Roger Lichtenberg. *Les momies et la mort en Égypte*. Paris: Terrance, 1998.

Dzierzykray-Rogalski, T. "Paleopathology of the Ptolemaic Inhabitants of Dakleh Oasis (Egypt)." *Journal of Human Evolution* 9 (1980): 71–74.

Ebbell, Bendix, ed. and trans. *The Papyrus Ebers: The Greatest Egyptian Medical Document*. Copenhagen: Levin and Munksgaard/London: Oxford University Press, 1937.

Ebers, Georg M., ed. *Papyros Ebers: Das hermetische Buch über die Arzeneimittel der alten Ägypter in hieratischer Schrift*. 2 vols. Leipzig: Englemann, 1875.

Edgerton, W. F. "The Strikes in Rameses III's Twenty-Ninth Year." *Journal of Near Eastern Studies* 10 (1951): 137–145.

El-Mahdy, Christine. *Momies, mythes et magie*. Trans. Christine Monnate and Marie Chemozay. Paris: Casterman, 1990.

Emery, Walter Bryan. *A Funerary Repast in an Egyptian Tomb of the Archaic Period*. Leiden: Nederlands Instituut voor het Nabije Oosten, 1962.

Engelbach, R., and D. E. Derry. "Mummification." *Annales du service des antiquités de l'Égypte* 4 (1942): 239–265.

Erman, Adolf. *Ägypten und ägyptisches Leben im Altertum*. Ed. Hermann Ranke. Tübingen: J. C. B. Mohr, 1923.

———. *Die Märchen des Papyrus Westcar*. Berlin: W. Spemann, 1890.

———. *La civilisation égyptienne dans l'antiquité*. Ed. Hermann Ranke. Trans. Charles Mathieu. Paris: Payot, 1985.

———. *The Literature of the Ancient Egyptians*. Trans. Aylward M. Blackman. London: Methuen, 1927.

Etaric, Ludovic. "L'alimentation et ses répercussions sur la sphère bucco-dentaire dans l'Égypte ancienne." Doctoral thesis in dental surgery, University of Paris V, 1998.

Ey, Henri. *Naissance de la médecine*. Paris: Masson, 1981.

Fage, Louis. *Commentaires sur la première Plaie d'Égypte*. Paris: Conférences du Palais de la découverte, 1953.

Falke, T. H., M. C. Zweypfenning, R. C. Zweypfenning, and A. E. James Jr. "Computed Tomography of an Ancient Egyptian." *Journal of Computer Assisted Tomography* 11 (1987): 745–747.

Faulkner, Raymond O. *A Concise Dictionary of Middle Egyptian*. Oxford: Oxford University Press, 1962.

Faure, C., and M. Bucaille. "Intérêt actuel de l'étude radiologique des momies pharaoniques." *Annales radiologiques* 19 (1976): 475–480.

Feldman, R. P., and J. T. Goodrich. "The Edwin Smith Surgical Papyrus." *Child's Nervous System* 15 (1999): 281–284.

Firchow, Otto, ed. *Aegyptologische Studien*. Berlin: Akademie-Verlag, 1955.

Fodor, J., J. C. Malott, and A. Y. King. "The Radiographic Investigation of Two Egyptian Mummies." *Radiologic Technology Journal* 54 (1983): 443–448.

Frommeyer, W. B., Jr. "Commentaries on the History of Medicine: From Primitive Medicine to the Hippocratic Era of Medicine." *Alabama Journal of Medical Science* 10 (1973): 340–348.

Gaafar, H., M. H. Abdel-Monem, and S. Elsheikh. "Nasal Endoscopy and CT Study of Pharaonic and Roman Mummies." *Acta Otolaryngolica* 119 (1999): 257–260.

Gabriel-Leroux, J. *Les premières civilisations de la Méditerranée*. Paris: Presses Universitaires de France, 1983.

Gardiner, Alan H. "The House of Life." *Journal of Egyptian Archaeology* 24 (1938): 157–179.

———. *The Kadesh Inscriptions of Ramesses II*. Oxford: Oxford University Press, 1960.

———. "Professional Magicians in Ancient Egypt." *Proceedings of the Society of Biblical Archeology* 39 (1917): 31–44.

———. *The Ramesseum Papyri.* Oxford: Oxford University Press, 1955.

———. *Royal Canon of Turin.* Oxford: Griffith Institute/Oxford University Press, 1959.

Gardiner, Alan H., T. Eric Peet, and Jaroslav Černý. *The Inscriptions of Sinai.* 2 vols. London: Egypt Exploration Society, 1952–1955.

Gemayel, Amin. *L'hygiène et la médecine à travers la Bible.* Paris: P. Geuthner, 1932.

Géraut, Christian, ed. *L'essentiel des pathologies professionnelles.* Paris: Ellipses, 1993.

Ghalioungui, Paul. "Four Landmarks of Egyptian Cardiology." *Journal of the Royal College of Physicians of London* 18 (1984): 182–186.

———. *The House of Life (Per Ankh): Magic and Medical Science in Ancient Egypt.* Amsterdam: B. M. Israël, 1973.

———. *La médecine des pharaons: magie et science médicale dans l'Égypte ancienne.* Paris: Laffont, 1983.

———. *Magic and Medical Science in Ancient Egypt.* London: Hodder and Stoughton, 1963.

———. *The Physicians of Pharaonic Egypt.* Cairo: Al-Ahram Center for Scientific Translation, 1983.

Ghalioungui, P., P. Khalil, and A. R. Ammar. "On an Ancient Egyptian Method of Diagnosing Pregnancy and Determining Foetal Sex." *Medical Historian* 7 (1963): 241–246.

Ghanem, A. N. "The Urology of Pharaonic Egypt." *British Journal of Urology* 85 (2000): 974.

Gispen, J. G. W. "Measuring the Patient in Ancient Egyptian Medical Texts." *Janus* 54 (1967): 224–227.

Glanville, S. R. K., ed. *The Legacy of Egypt.* Oxford: Clarendon Press, 1942.

Godron, G. "Notes sur l'histoire de la médecine et l'occupation perse en Égypte." In *Hommage à François Daumas,* 285–287. Montpellier: Publications de l'Université de Montpellier, 1986.

Goyon, Jean-Claude. *Le papyrus du Louvre n° 3279.* Cairo: Institut Français d'Archéologie Orientale, 1966.

Goyon, Jean-Claude, and Patrice Josset. *Un corps pour l'éternité: autopsie d'une momie.* Paris: Le Léopard d'Or, 1988.

Grandet, Pierre, ed. and trans. *Hymnes de la religion d'Aton: hymnes du XIVe siècle avant J.-C.* Paris: Seuil, 1995.

———. "La communauté d'artisans de Deir el-Medineh sous les Ramsès." In *Les artistes de pharaon,* 43–47. Paris: Éditions de la Réunion des Musées Nationaux, 2002.

Granville, A. B. "An Essay on Egyptian Mummies with Observations on the

Art of Embalming among the Ancient Egyptians." *Philosophical Transactions of the Royal Society* 115 (1825): 219–319.

Grapow, Hermann, Hildegard von Deines, and Wolfhart Westendorf, eds. and trans. *Grundriss der Medizin der alten Ägypter.* 9 vols. Berlin: Akademie Verlag, 1954–1973.

Gray, P. H. "Radiography of Ancient Egyptian Mummies." *Medical Radiography and Photography* 43 (1967): 34–44.

Griffith, Francis Ll. *The Petrie Papyri: Hieratic Papyri from Kahun and Gurob (Principally of the Middle Kingdom).* 2 vols. London: Bernard Quaritch, 1898.

Griffith, Francis Ll., and Herbert Thompson. *The Demotic Magical Papyrus of London and Leiden.* 3 vols. London: H. Grevel, 1904–1909.

Grossman, E. A., and N. A. Posner. "The Circumcision Controversy: An Update." *Obstetrics and Gynecology Annual* 13 (1984): 181–195.

Guest, E. M. "Ancient Egyptian Physicians." *British Medical Journal* 1 (1926): 706.

Guiart, Jules. "L'obstétrique dans l'ancienne Égypte." In *Acte du 2ᵉ congrès international d'histoire de la médecine* (Évreux: Herissey, 1922), 54–63.

Gunn, B. "Interpreters of Dreams in Ancient Egypt." *Journal of Egyptian Archaeology* 4 (1917): 252.

Hamarneh, S. K. "Excavated Surgical Instruments from Old Cairo, Egypt." *Annali dell'Istituto e Museo di Storia della Scienza di Firenze* 2 (1977): 3–14.

Harwood-Nash, D. C. "Computed Tomography of Ancient Egyptian Mummies." *Journal of Computer Assisted Tomography* 3 (1979): 768–773.

Hauben, D. J., and G. J. Sonneveld. "The Influence of War on the Development of Plastic Surgery." *Annals of Plastic Surgery* 10 (1983): 65–69.

Hedges, R. E. M., and B. A. Sykes. "The Extraction and Isolation of DNA from Archeological Bone." In Davies and Walker, eds., *Biological Anthropology and the Study of Ancient Egypt,* 98–103.

Helck, W. "Eine Briefsammlung aus der Verwaltung des Amuntemples." *Journal of the American Research Center in Egypt* 6 (1967): 135–151.

Hennequin, Pascal. "Santé et hygiène de l'enfant dans l'Égypte ancienne." Doctoral thesis in medicine, University of Nancy, 2001.

Henrion, Laurence. "L'athérosclérose dans l'Égypte ancienne." Doctoral thesis in medicine, University of Nancy I, 1997.

Herodotus. Trans. A. D. Godley. Loeb Classical Library, 4 vols. Cambridge, Mass.: Harvard University Press, 1921–1924.

———. *The Histories.* Trans. Aubrey de Sélincourt, rev. with introductory matter and notes by John Marincola. New York: Penguin, 1996.

————. *Oeuvres complètes*. Trans. Andrée Barguet. Paris: Gallimard/
Bibliothèque de la Pléiade, 1964.

Hieratic Papyri in the British Museum. 3rd series, nos. 53–54. London: Department of Egyptian and Assyrian Antiquities, British Museum, 1935.

Hill, B., I. Macleod, and L. Watson. "Facial Reconstruction of a 3500-Year-
Old Egyptian Mummy Using Axial Computed Tomography." *Journal of
Audiovisual Media in Medicine* 16 (1993): 11–13.

Hippocrates. Trans. W. H. S. Jones et al. Loeb Classical Library, 8 vols.
Cambridge, Mass.: Harvard University Press, 1984–1994.

Homer. *The Odyssey*. Trans. A. T. Murray, rev. George E. Dimock. Loeb Classical Library, 2 vols. Cambridge, Mass.: Harvard University Press, 1998.

Horne, P. D., and P. K. Lewin. "Autopsy of an Egyptian Mummy: Electron
Microscopy of Mummified Tissue." *Canadian Medical Association
Journal* 117 (1977): 472–473.

Horne, P. D., and D. S. Redford. "Aspergillosis and Dracunculosis in
Mummies from the Tomb of Parennefer." *Paleopathology Newsletter* 92
(1995): 10–12.

Hornung, Erik. *L'esprit au temps des pharaons*. Trans. Michèle Hulin. Paris:
Hachette, 1998. In English, *Idea into Image: Essays on Ancient Egyptian
Thought*. Trans. Elizabeth Bredeck. New York: Timken, 1992.

Hulse, E. V. "Leprosy and Ancient Egypt." *Lancet* 11 (1972): 1024–1025.

Iles, J. D. "Autopsy of an Egyptian Mummy (Nakht-ROM 1)." *Canadian
Medical Association Journal* 118 (1978): 20–21.

Iversen, Erik. *The Myth of Egypt and Its Hieroglyphics in European Tradition*.
Copenhagen: Gad, 1961.

————, ed. *Papyrus Carlsberg No. VIII, with Some Remarks on the Egyptian
Origin of Some Popular Birth Prognoses*. Copenhagen: Munksgaard,
1939.

Janssen, Jac J. "Absence from Work by the Necropolis Workmen of Thebes."
Studien zur Altägyptischen Kultur 8 (1980): 127–152.

————. *Commodity Prices from the Ramessid Period: An Economic Study of
the Village of Necropolis Workmen at Thebes*. Leiden: Brill, 1975.

Janssen, Rosalind, and Jac J. Janssen. *Growing Up in Ancient Egypt*. London:
Rubicon Press, 1990.

Jonckheere, Frans. "À la recherche du chirurgien égyptien." *Chronique
d'Égypte* 26 (1951): 28–45.

————. "Considération sur l'auxillaire médical pharaonique." *Chronique
d'Égypte* 28 (1953): 62–65.

————. "La place du prêtre de Sekhmet dans le corps médical de l'ancienne
Égypte." *Archives internationales d'histoire des sciences* 4 (1951): 915–
924.

————. "Le cadre professionel et administratif des médecins égyptiens." *Chronique d'Égypte* 26 (1951): 237–268.

————. "Le monde des malades dans les textes non médicaux." *Chronique d'Égypte* 25 (1950): 213–232.

————. "Le 'préparateur de remèdes' dans l'organisation de la pharmacie égyptienne." In Firchow, ed., *Aegyptologische Studien*, 149–161.

————. *Les médecins de l'Égypte pharaonique: essai de prosographie.* Brussels: Fondation Égyptologique Reine Élisabeth, 1958.

————. "Un chapître de pédiatrie égyptienne: l'allaitement." *Aesculape* 36 (1955): 203–223.

Jouanna, Jacques. *Hippocrates.* Trans. M. B. DeBevoise. Baltimore: Johns Hopkins University Press, 1999.

Känel, Frédérique von. *Les prêtres-ouâb de Sekhmet et les conjurateurs de Serket.* Paris: Presses Universitaires de France, 1984.

Kitchen, K. A. *Pharaoh Triumphant: The Life and Times of Rameses II, King of Egypt.* Warminster, England: Aris and Phillips, 1983.

Knoeller, S. M., and C. Seifried. "Historical Perspective: History of Spinal Surgery." *Spine* 25 (2000): 2838–2843.

Koenig, H. G. "Religion and Medicine I: Historical Background and Reasons for Separation." *International Journal of Psychiatry* 30 (2000): 385–398.

Koenig, Yvan. *Magie et magiciens dans l'Égypte ancienne.* Paris: Pygmalion, 1994.

Koller, J., U. Baumer, Y. Kaup, H. Etspuler, and U. Weser. "Embalming Was Used in Old Kingdom." *Nature* 391 (1998): 343–344.

Lalouette, Claire. *Au royaume d'Égypte: le temps des rois-dieux.* Paris: Fayard, 1991.

————. *Textes sacrés et textes profanes de l'ancienne Égypte: traductions et commentaires.* Paris: Gallimard, 1984.

Leavesley, J. H. "Akhenaten." *Medical Journal of Australia* 142 (1985): 475–484.

Leca, Ange Pierre. *La médecine égyptienne au temps des pharaons.* Paris: Dacosta, 1983.

————. *Les momies.* Paris: Hachette, 1976.

Leek, F. F. "Observations on a Collection of Crania from the Mastabas of the Reign of Cheops at Giza." *Journal of Egyptian Archeology* 66 (1980): 36–45.

————. "Teeth and Bread in Ancient Egypt." *Journal of Egyptian Archeology* 58 (1972): 126–132.

Lefebvre, Gustave. *Essai sur la médecine égyptienne de l'époque pharaonique.* Paris: Presses Universitaires de France, 1956.

Lerman, Charles. "L'école de médecine d'Alexandrie." Doctoral thesis in medicine. Faculté de Médecine Saint-Louis-Lariboisière, Paris, 1980.

Lethor, Jean-Paul. "Du coeur et des vaisseaux dans l'Égypte ancienne: étude de textes, étude de momies." Doctoral thesis in medicine, University of Nancy I, 1989.

Levin, S. "Death of the First-Born: The Tenth Plague." *South African Medical Journal* 48 (1974): 1038–1042.

Lexa, František. *La magie dans l'Égypte antique.* Paris: Paul Geuthner, 1925.

———. *Papyrus Insinger: les enseignements moraux d'un scribe égyptien du premier siècle après J.-C.* Paris: Paul Geuthner, 1926.

Libby, Willard F. *Radiocarbon Dating.* Chicago: University of Chicago Press, 1952.

Lichtenthaeler, Charles. *Histoire de la médecine.* Paris: Fayard, 1978.

Lichtheim, Miriam. *Late Egyptian Wisdom Literature in the International Context: A Study of Demotic Instructions.* Freiburg: Universitätsverlag, 1983.

Lloyd, Alan B. "The Late Period." In Shaw, ed., *Oxford History of Ancient Egypt,* 369–394.

Lucas, Alfred, and J. R. Harris. *Ancient Egyptian Materials and Industries.* 4th rev. ed. London: E. Arnold, 1962.

Lucian of Samosata. Trans. A. M. Harmon. Loeb Classical Library, 8 vols. Cambridge, Mass.: Harvard University Press, 1960–1967.

Malek, Jaromir. *Egypt: 4000 Years of Art.* London: Phaidon, 2003.

Manialawy, M., and R. Meligny. "Endoscopic Examination of Egyptian Mummies." *Endoscopy* 10 (1978): 191–194.

Mannliche, Lise. *An Ancient Egyptian Herbal.* London: British Museum Publications, 1989.

Marion, L. R. "Dentistry of Ancient Egypt." *Journal of the History of Dentistry* 44 (1996): 15–17.

Marota, I., and F. Rollo. "Molecular Paleontology." *Cellular and Molecular Life Sciences* 59 (2002): 97–111.

Martinez, Philippe. *Égypte.* Paris: Liana Levi, 1999.

Martiny, Marcel. *Hippocrate et la médecine.* Paris: Fayard, 1964.

Marx, M., and S. H. D'Auria. "CT Examination of Eleven Egyptian Mummies." *Radiographics* 6 (1986): 321–330.

———. "Three-Dimensional CT Reconstructions of an Ancient Human Egyptian Mummy." *American Journal of Roentgenology* 150 (1988): 147–149.

Masali, M., and B. Chiarelli. "Demographic Data on the Remains of Ancient Egyptians." In *Population Biology of the Ancient Egyptians,* ed. Don R. Brothwell and B. A. Chiarelli (London: Academic Press, 1973), 161–169.

Maspero, Gaston, ed. *Études de mythologie et d'archéologie égyptienne.* 8 vols. Paris: E. Leroux, 1893–1916.

———. *Le papyrus Ebers et la médecine égyptienne.* Paris: Ernest Leroux, 1898.

Massart, Adhémar. *The Leiden Magical Papyrus I 343 and I 345.* Leiden: E. J. Brill, 1954.

Mazzone, P., M. A. Banchero, and S. Esposito. "Neurological Sciences at Their Origin: Neurology and Neurological Surgery in the Medicine of Ancient Egypt." *Pathologica* 79 (1987): 787–800.

"Le médecin de pharaon." *Sciences et avenir* 662 (April 2002): 32–34.

Meeks, D. "Notes de lexicographies." *Bulletin de l'Institut français d'archéologie orientale* 77 (1977): 87–88.

Menard, Guillaume-Pierre. "Les techniques chirurgicales dans l'antiquité égyptienne." Doctoral thesis in medicine, University of Lyons I, 1991.

Merkle, E. M., F. Parsche, J. J. Vogel, H. S. Brambs, and W. Pirsig. "Computed Tomographic Measurements of the Nasal Sinuses and Frontal Bone in Mummy Heads Artificially Deformed in Infancy." *American Journal of Rhinology* 12 (1998): 99–104.

Miller, R., D. D. Callas, S. E. Kahn, V. Ricchiati, and F. Apple. "Evidence of Myocardial Infarction in Mummified Human Tissue." *Journal of the American Medical Association* 284 (2000): 831–832.

Miller, R. L., S. Ikram, G. J. Armelagos, R. Walker, W. B. Harer, C. S. Schiff, D. Baggett, M. Carrigan, and S. M. Maret. "Diagnosis of *Plasmodium falciparum* Infections in Mummies Using the Rapid Manual *Para*Sight™-F Test." *Transactions of the Royal Society of Tropical Medicine and Hygiene* 88 (1994): 31–32.

Millo, Lionel. "La mort chez les Égyptiens." Doctoral thesis in medicine, University of Aix-Marseille II, 1992.

Montserrat, Dominic. *Akhenaten: History, Fantasy, and Ancient Egypt.* London: Routledge, 2000.

Moodie, Roy Lee. *Roentgenologic Studies of Egyptian and Peruvian Mummies.* Chicago: Field Museum of Natural History, 1931.

Moore, N. "Drugs in Ancient Populations," *Lancet* 341 (1993): 1157.

Morenz, Siegfried. *La religion égyptienne.* Trans. Laurent Jospin. Paris: Payot, 1984. Translation of Morenz, *Ägyptische Religion* (Stuttgart: W. Kohlhammer, 1960). In English, *Egyptian Religion,* trans. Ann E. Keep (Ithaca: Cornell University Press, 1992).

Morice, Philippe. "La gynécologie et l'obstétrique en Égypte pharaonique." Doctoral thesis in medicine, University of Paris-V, 1992.

Morice, P., P. Josset, and J.-C. Colau. "Gynécologie et obstétrique dans l'ancienne Égypte." *Journal de gynécologie obstétrique et biologie de la reproduction* 23 (1994): 131–136.

Morse, D., D. R. Brothwell, and P. J. Ucko. "Tuberculosis in Ancient Egypt." *American Review of Respiratory Diseases* 90 (1964): 524–541.

Moutet, Daniel. "Fossoyeurs et services funéraires." In Géraut, ed., *L'essentiel des pathologies professionnelles.*

Murray, Mary Ann. "Fruits, Vegetables, Pulses, and Condiments." In Nicholson and Shaw, eds., *Ancient Egyptian Materials and Technology,* 609–655.

Nanetti, O. "Ricerche sui medici e sulla medecina nei papiri." *Aegyptus* 21 (1941): 304–314.

Newberry, P. E., ed. *The Amherst Papyri, Being an Account of the Egyptian Papyri in the Collection of the Right Hon. Lord Amherst of Hackney, F.S.A. at Didlington Hall, Norfolk.* London, 1899.

Nicholson, Paul T., and Ian Shaw, eds. *Ancient Egyptian Materials and Technology.* Cambridge: Cambridge University Press, 2000.

Nickol, T., R. Germer, S. Lieberenz, F. Schmidt, and W. Wilke. "An Examination of the Dental State of an Egyptian Mummy by Means of Computer Tomography: A Contribution to 'Dentistry in Ancient Egypt.'" *Journal of the History of Dentistry* 43 (1995): 105–112.

Nof, D., and N. Paldor. "Are There Oceanographic Explanations for the Israelites' Crossing of the Red Sea?" *Bulletin of the American Meteorological Society* 73 (1992): 1305–1314.

Notman, Derek N. H. "Ancient Scannings: Computed Tomography of Egyptian Mummies." In David, ed., *Science in Egyptology,* 251–320.

Notman, D. N. H., J. Tashjian, A. C. Aufderheide, O. W. Cass, O. C. Shane 3rd, T. H. Berquist, J. E. Gray, and E. Gedgaudas. "Modern Imaging and Endoscopic Biopsy Techniques in Egyptian Mummies." *American Journal of Roentgenology* 146 (1986): 93–96.

Nunn, John F. *Ancient Egyptian Medicine.* London: British Museum Press/Norman: University of Oklahoma Press, 1996.

Nunn, J. F., and C. N. Andrew. "Egyptian Antiquities at the Royal College of Surgeons of England." *Annals of the Royal College of Surgeons of England* 59 (1977): 342–347.

Pääbo, S. "Molecular Cloning of Ancient Egyptian Mummy DNA." *Nature* 314 (1985): 644–645.

———. "Preservation of DNA in Ancient Egyptian Mummies." *Journal of Archeological Science* 12 (1985): 411–417.

Pahl, Wolfgang M. "Possibilities, Limitations, and Prospects of Computed Tomography as a Non-Invasive Method of Mummy Studies." In David, ed., *Science in Egyptology,* 13–24.

———. "La tomographie par ordinateur appliquée aux momies égyptiennes." *Bulletins et mémoires de la Société d'anthropologie de Paris* 13 (1981): 343–356.

Panagiotakopulu, E. "Pharaonic Egypt and the Origins of Plague." *Journal of Biogeography* 31 (2004): 269–274.

Peacock, David. "The Roman Period." In Shaw, ed., *Oxford History of Ancient Egypt,* 427–428.

Peet, T. Eric. *The Great Tomb Robberies of the Twentieth Egyptian Dynasty.* Oxford: Clarendon Press, 1930.

Perrin, C., V. Noly, R. Mourer, and D. Schmitt. "Préservation des structures cutanées des momies égyptiennes." *Annales de dermatologie et de vénérologie* 121 (1994): 470–475.

Petrie, W. M. Flinders. *The Royal Tombs of the First Dynasty.* 2 vols. London: Egypt Exploration Fund, 1900–1901.

———. *Tools and Weapons.* London: Constable, 1917.

Picard, Rémi. "La médecine magique dans l'Égypte ancienne: notions fondamentales et concepts neuropsychiatriques." Doctoral thesis in medicine, University of Aix-Marseille II, 1999.

Piepenbrink, D., J. Frahm, A. Haase, and D. Matthaei. "Nuclear Magnetic Resonance Imaging of Mummified Corpses." *American Journal of Physical Anthropology* 70 (1986): 27–28.

Pleyte, Willem, and Francesco Rossi, eds. *Papyrus de Turin.* 2 vols. Leiden: E. J. Brill, 1869–1876.

Pliny the Elder. *Natural History.* Trans. H. Rackham and W. H. S. Jones. Loeb Classical Library, 10 vols. Cambridge, Mass.: Harvard University Press, 1938–1963.

Posener, G. "L'attribution d'un nom à l'enfant." *Revue d'égyptologie* 22 (1970): 20–25.

Posener, Georges, Serge Sauneron, and Jean Yoyotte. *Dictionnaire de la civilisation égyptienne,* rev. ed. Paris: Fernand Hazan, 1986.

Préaux, C. "Les prescriptions médicales des ostracas grecs de la bibliothèque Bodléenne." *Chronique d'Égypte* 35 (1956): 135–148.

Pretre Guignard, Dominique. "Conditions de travail dans l'Égypte ancienne vues sous l'angle de la médecine du travail." Doctoral thesis in medicine, University of Nantes, 1993.

Puech, P.-F. "Autopsie d'une momie égyptienne." *Nouvelles archives du Museum d'histoire naturelle de Lyon* 25 (1987).

Quenouille, J.-J. "L'art dentaire dans l'Égypte ancienne." *Information dentaire* 27 (1977): 25–38.

Rachet, Guy. *Dictionnaire de la civilisation égyptienne.* Paris: Larousse, 1998.

Ray, J.-J. "Papyrus Carlsberg 67: A Healing Prayer from the Fayum." *Journal of Egyptian Archaeology* 61 (1975): 181–188.

Ray, John. *Reflections of Osiris: Lives from Ancient Egypt.* Oxford: Oxford University Press, 2002.

Redford, Donald B., ed. *The Ancient Gods Speak: A Guide to Ancient Religion.* New York: Oxford University Press, 2002.

———, ed. *Oxford Encyclopedia of Ancient Egypt.* 3 vols. Oxford: Oxford University Press, 2001.

Reisner, George A., ed. *The Hearst Medical Papyrus.* Leipzig: Hinrichs, 1905.

Remondon, R. "Problèmes de bilinguisme dans l'Égypte lagide (UPZ, I, 48)." *Chronique d'Égypte* 39 (1964): 126–146.

Revelat, Daniel. "Pensées et pratiques médicales de l'Égypte pharaonique." Doctoral thesis in medicine, University of Nice, 1984.

Reyman, T. A. "Les momies égyptiennes." *La recherche* 14 (1984): 792–799.

Reyman, T. A., M. R. Zimmerman, and P. K. Lewin. "Autopsy of an Egyptian Mummy: A Histological Investigation." *Canadian Medical Association Journal* 117 (1977): 470–472.

Reymond, E. A. E. *From the Contents of the Libraries of the Suchos Temples in the Fayyum: A Medical Book from Crocodilopolis, P. Vindob. D. 6257.* Vienna: Hollinek, 1976.

Riad, Naguib. *La médecine au temps des pharaons.* Paris: Maloine, 1955.

Riginos, Alice Swift. *Platonica: The Anecdotes concerning the Life and Teachings of Plato.* Leiden: E. J. Brill, 1976.

Rinelli, Marie-Étienne. "Diagnostic exacte de la dysmorphie du Pharaon Amenophis IV dit Akhenaton." Doctoral thesis in medicine, Faculté Cochin-Port Royal, Paris, 1988.

Risse, G. B. "Pharaoh Akhenaten of Ancient Egypt: Controversies among Egyptologists and Physicians regarding His Postulated Illness." *Journal of the History of Medicine and Allied Sciences* 26 (1971): 3–17.

———. "Rational Egyptian Surgery: A Cranial Injury Discussed in the Edwin Smith Papyrus." *Bulletin of the New York Academy of Medicine* 48 (1972): 912–919.

Ritner, Robert K. "Magic in Medicine." In Redford, ed., *Oxford Encyclopedia of Ancient Egypt,* 2:326–329.

———. "Medicine." In Redford, ed., *Oxford Encyclopedia of Ancient Egypt,* 2:353–356.

Romant, Bernard. *La vie en Égypte aux temps antiques.* Paris: Minerva, 1982.

Rose, Jerome C., George J. Armelagos, and L. Stephen Perry. "Dental Anthropology of the Nile Valley." In Davies and Walker, eds., *Biological Anthropology and the Study of Ancient Egypt,* 61–74.

Ruffer, Marc Armand. *Studies in the Paleopathology of Egypt.* Ed. Roy L. Moodie. Chicago: University of Chicago Press, 1921.

Saint-Hilaire, Geoffroy. "Note sur un monstre humain trouvé dans les ruines de Thèbes." *Bulletin des sciences médicales et archives générales de médecine* 8 (1826): 105.

Salem, M. E., and G. Eknoyan. "The Kidney in Ancient Egyptian Medicine: Where Does It Stand?" *American Journal of Nephrology* 19 (1999): 140–147.

Samuel, D. "Cereal Foods and Nutrition in Ancient Egypt." *Nutrition* 13 (1997): 579–580.

Sanchez, G. M. "A Neurosurgeon's View of the Battle Reliefs of King Sety I:

Aspects of Neurological Importance." *Journal of the American Research Center in Egypt* 37 (2000): 143–165.

———. "Injuries in the Battle of Kadesh." *KMT: A Modern Journal of Ancient Egypt* 14 (2003): 58–65.

Sandford, M. K., and G. E. Kissling. "Multivariate Analysis of Elemental Hair Concentrations from a Medieval Nubian Population." *American Journal of Physical Anthropology* 95 (1994): 41–52.

Sandison, A. T. "The Histological Examination of Mummified Material." *Stain Technology* 30 (1955): 277–283.

Sarazin, Olivier. "La pathologie cardio-vasculaire dans l'Égypte ancienne." Doctoral thesis in medicine, Créteil-University of Paris-XII, 2001.

Sauneron, Serge. "À propos d'un prognostic de naissance: Papyrus de Berlin 3038." *Bulletin de l'Institut français d'archéologie orientale* 59 (1960): 29–30.

———. "Les dix mois précédents la naissance." *Bulletin de l'Institut français d'archéologie orientale* 58 (1959): 33–34.

———. *Les prêtres de l'ancienne Égypte.* 2d ed. Paris: Perséa, 1988.

———. "Une conception anatomique tardive." *Bulletin de l'Institut français d'archéologie orientale* 51 (1952): 51–62.

———. *Un traité égyptien d'ophiologie: papyrus du Brooklyn Museum n° 47.218.48 et .85.* Cairo: L'Institut Français d'Archéologie Orientale, 1989.

Scarborough, J. "On Medications for Burns in Classical Antiquity." *Clinical Plastic Surgery* 10 (1983): 603–610.

Schwartz, J.-C. "La médecine dentaire dans l'Égypte pharaonique." *Bulletin de la Société égyptologique de Genève* 2 (1979): 37–43.

Shampo, M. A., and R. A. Kyle. "Medical Mythology: Horus." *Mayo Clinic Proceedings* 67 (1992): 36.

Shattock, S. G. "Minutes of a Meeting of the Pathological Section of the Royal Society of Medicine ('Microscopic Sections of the Aorta of King Meneptah')." *Lancet* (30 January 1909): 319.

Shaw, Ian, ed. *Oxford History of Ancient Egypt.* Oxford: Oxford University Press, 2000.

Sigerist, Henry E. *A History of Medicine,* vol. 1: *Primitive and Archaic Medicine.* New York: Oxford University Press, 1951.

Simpson, William Kelly. "Instructions of Khety." In Redford, ed., *Oxford Encyclopedia of Ancient Egypt,* 2:174–175.

Sluglett, J. "Mummification in Ancient Egypt." *West of England Medical Journal* 104 (1990): 117–119.

Smith, G. Elliot, and Warren R. Dawson. *Egyptian Mummies.* London: Allen and Unwin, 1924.

Smith, G. Elliot, and D. E. Derry. "Anatomical Report." In *Archeological Survey of Nubia: Bulletin 6* (Cairo: National Printing Department, 1910).

Spaeth, Dominique. "Pneumologie et cancérologie dans la médecine de l'Égypte à travers les écrits médicaux, l'art et les données de la paléopathologie." Doctoral thesis in medicine, University of Nancy, 1990.

Staden, Heinrich von. *Herophilus: The Art of Medicine in Early Alexandria.* Cambridge: Cambridge University Press, 1989.

Steuer, R. O. "Whdw: Aetiological Principle of Pyaemia in Ancient Egyptian Medicine." *Bulletin of the History of Medicine,* supplement 10 (1948).

Steuer, Robert O., and J. B. de C. M. Saunders. *Ancient Egyptian and Cnidean Medicine.* Berkeley: University of California Press, 1959.

Stevens, J. M. "Gynaecology from Ancient Egypt: The Papyrus Kahun." *Medical Journal of Australia* 2 (1975): 949–952.

Strouhal, Eugen. *Life in Ancient Egypt.* Trans. Deryck Viney. Cambridge: Cambridge University Press, 1992.

Sullivan, R. "Divine and Rational: The Reproductive Health of Women in Ancient Egypt." *Obstetrical and Gynecological Survey* 52 (1997): 635–642.

———. "The Identity and Work of the Ancient Egyptian Surgeon." *Journal of the Royal Society of Medicine* 89 (1996): 467–473.

Suys, Émile. *La sagesse d'Ani: texte, traduction et commentaires.* Rome: Pontifico Istituto, 1935.

———. [The Vatican Papyrus.] *Orientalia* (new series) 3 (1934): 68–87.

Tapp, Eddie. "Disease in the Manchester Mummies." In David, ed., *Manchester Museum Mummy Project,* 95–102.

———. "The Unwrapping of 1770." In David, ed., *Science in Egyptology,* 51–56.

Thekkaniyil, J. K., S. E. Bishara, and M. A. James. "Dental and Skeletal Findings on an Ancient Egyptian Mummy." *American Journal of Orthodontics and Dentofacial Orthopedics* 117 (2000): 10–14.

Théma: Encyclopédie Larousse, vol. 1: *Les hommes et leur histoire.* Paris: Larousse, 1990.

Thorwald, Jürgen. *Histoire de la médecine dans l'antiquité.* Trans. Henri Daussy. Paris: Hachette, 1966.

Trémillon, Sylvie. "Essai d'interprétation des plaies d'Égypte." Doctoral thesis in medicine, Paris XI-Kremlin Bicêtre, 1989.

Vercoutter, Jean. *À la recherche de l'Égypte oubliée.* Paris: Gallimard, 1986.

———. *Essai sur les relations entre Égyptiens et Préhellènes.* Paris: A. Maisonneuve, 1954.

Vikentieff, V. "Deux rites du jubilé royal à l'époque protodynastique." *Bulletin de l'Institut d'Égypte* 32 (1949–1950): 171–228.

Viso, L., and J. Uriach. "The 'Guardians of the Anus' and Their Practice." *International Journal of Colorectal Disease* 10 (1995): 229–231.

Volten, Aksel, ed. *Demotische Traumdeutung (Pap. Carlsberg XIII und XIV verso).* Copenhagen: Munksgaard, 1942.

Walle, R. van de, and H. de Meulenaere. "Compléments à la prosographie médicale." *Revue d'égyptologie* 25 (1973): 58–83.

Waszak, S. J. "The Historic Significance of Circumcision." *Obstetrics and Gynecology* 51 (1978): 499–501.

Weeks, Kent R. "The Anatomical Knowledge of the Ancient Egyptians and the Representation of the Human Figure in Egyptian Art." Ph.D. thesis, Yale University, 1970.

Weigall, A. "The Mummy of Akhenaten." *Journal of Egyptian Archeology* 8 (1922): 193–199.

Weill, R. "Les transmissions littéraires d'Égypte à Israël." *Revue d'égyptologie* (1950).

Wein, S. "The Plagues of Egypt: What Killed the Animals and the First-Born?" *Medical Journal of Australia* 159 (1993): 285–286.

Weinberger, B. W. "The Dental Art in Ancient Egypt." *Journal of the American Dental Association* 34 (1947): 170–184.

Willerson, J. T., and R. Teaff. "Egyptian Contributions to Cardiovascular Medicine." *Texas Heart Institute Journal* 23 (1996): 191–200.

Wiltse, L. L., and T. G. Pait. "Herophilus of Alexandria (325–255 B.C.): The Father of Anatomy." *Spine* 23 (1998): 1904–1919.

Winter, Alain. "L'hygiène dans l'Égypte pharaonique." Doctoral thesis in medicine, Faculté Cochin-Port Royal, Paris, 1972.

Wolf, G. "A Historical Note on the Mode of Administration of Vitamin A for the Cure of Night Blindness." *American Journal of Clinical Nutrition* 31 (1978): 290–292.

Woodward, T. E. "Religion and Medicine: An Ancient Relationship." *Maryland Medical Journal* 38 (1989): 568–572.

Wreszinski, Walter, ed. *Der grosse medizinische Papyrus des Berliner Museums (Pap. Berl. 3038)*. Leipzig: Hinrichs, 1909.

———. *Der Londoner medizinische Papyrus (Brit. Museum nr. 10,059) und der Papyrus Hearst in Transkription: Übersetzung und Kommentar.* Leipzig: Hinrichs, 1912.

———. *Der Papyrus Ebers: Umschrift, Übersetzung und Kommentar.* Leipzig: Hinrichs, 1913.

Yahuda, A. S. "Medical and Anatomical Terms in the Pentateuch in the Light of Egyptian Medical Papyri." *Journal of the History of Medicine and Allied Sciences* 2 (1947): 549–574.

Yoyotte, J. "Une théorie étiologique des médecins égyptiens." *Kêmi* 18 (1968): 79–84.

Žába, Zybněk, ed. and trans. *Les maximes de Ptahhotep*. Prague: Éditions de l'Académie tchécoslovaque des sciences, 1956.

Zimmerman, M. R. "The Paleopathology of the Cardiovascular System." *Texas Heart Institute Journal* 20 (1993): 252–257.

Zumla, A., and A. Lulat. "Honey: A Remedy Rediscovered." *Journal of the Royal Society of Medicine* 82 (1989): 384–385.

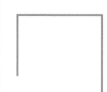

Illustration Credits

page 54

The mummy of Rameses II. Egyptian Museum, Cairo. © Scala/Art Resource, New York

page 57

Rosalie David and her team. Courtesy Rosalie David

page 58

Mummy being placed in a CAT scanner. Photograph by Eric Workman for the Museum of Science, Boston

page 73

Wooden amulet showing a mother and her newborn. British Museum. © Werner Forman/Art Resource, New York

page 80

Lactation bottle. Courtesy Rosicrucian Egyptian Museum, San Jose, California

page 83

Bas-relief from the tomb of Haremheb at Biban el-Muluk. Rijksmuseum van Oudheden, Leiden. © Erich Lessing/Art Resource, New York

page 91

Scene from a relief in the tomb of Ankhmahor at Saqqara. © Werner Forman/Art Resource, New York

page 98

Limestone bas-relief of Rameses II. The Louvre, Paris. © Erich Lessing/ Art Resource, New York

page 105

The "Polio stele." Courtesy Glyptotek Museum, Copenhagen

page 107

The queen of Punt. Egyptian Museum, Cairo. © Erich Lessing/Art Resource, New York

page 108

Akhenaten making an offering to Aten. Painted limestone stele. © Scala/ Art Resource, New York

page 111

Wallpainting showing a blind harpist. © Erich Lessing/Art Resource, New York

page 117

Painted limestone relief of a hippopotamus hunt. Staatliche Museen zu Berlin. © Margarete Buesing/Bildarchiv Preussischer Kulturbesitz/ Art Resource, New York

page 120

Wallpainting showing a farmer plowing his field while his wife sows seed.
© Erich Lessing/Art Resource, New York

page 122

Papyrus used as a talisman against fever. The Louvre, Paris. © Erich Lessing/
Art Resource, New York

page 124

Detail of a wallpainting in the tomb of Mennah. © Erich Lessing/
Art Resource, New York

page 125

Carved relief from the base of the pyramid of Unas. © Erich Lessing/
Art Resource, New York

page 133

Carpenters, sculptors, and stonecutters. From the tomb of Mereruka at
Saqqara. © Werner Forman/Art Resource, New York

page 134

Linked wooden vessels that contained cosmetic preparations and ointments.
The Louvre, Paris. © Werner Forman/Art Resource, New York

page 136

Wallpainting from the tomb of Rekhmere, in the cemetery of Sheikh Abd
al-Qurnah in Thebes. © Erich Lessing/Art Resource, New York

page 138

Stele listing spells to protect against venomous bites. Courtesy The
Metropolitan Museum of Art, Fletcher Fund, 1950 (50.85). Photograph
© 1993 The Metropolitan Museum of Art

page 142

Cippus of Horus. Courtesy Museum of Fine Arts, Boston

page 146

Wallpainting of military life from the tomb of Userhet. © Werner Forman/
Art Resource, New York

page 151

Scene from the tomb of Senet and Khety. © Erich Lessing/Art Resource,
New York

page 153

Relief from the mortuary temple of Rameses II at Thebes. © Erich Lessing/
Art Resource, New York

page 156

Raphael's fresco of the parting of the Red Sea. Vatican Palace, Rome.
© Scala/Art Resource, New York

page 159

Wooden figurines from a tomb shown grinding grain, kneading dough, and shaping and cooking bread. Museo Egizio, Turin. © Erich Lessing/Art Resource, New York

page 162

Wallpainting from the tomb of Inherka in Deir el-Medina. © Borromeo/Art Resource, New York

page 166

A slave being beaten by an overseer, from the tomb of Mennah. © Erich Lessing/Art Resource, New York

page 170

Painted limestone figure of a scribe. The Louvre, Paris. © Erich Lessing/Art Resource

page 176

Limestone painting of an acrobatic female dancer. Museo Egizio, Turin. © Alinari/Art Resource, New York

Acknowledgments

We would like first of all to thank our wives, Fanny and Corinne, for their invaluable support and complete understanding, without which this long and meticulous joint undertaking would not have been possible. We also thank for their support Salomé, Bethsabée, and Naomie, to whom their fathers and grandfather have sought to transmit their enthusiasm for ancient Egypt.

We owe a special debt of gratitude to Daniel Soulié at the École du Louvre, who kindly reviewed an earlier version of the book and gave us the benefit of his learning and sensible advice, and to Dr. Thierry Bardinet, who so generously shared the fruits of his exceptional achievement in translating the medical papyri.

We extend our gratitude as well to Sylvie Gillet, Sylvie Mouchès, and Fabienne Dumontet, who patiently and efficiently helped turn our manuscript into a book. And to Liana Levi, without whose continuing support and encouragement neither of us would have had the courage to see this work through to its conclusion.

Our thanks are due as well to Dr. Patrice Josset, who responded warmly to the idea of writing such a book in the first place; to Patrick Conan, at the Centre de Documentation d'Histoire de la Médecine in the University of Paris-VI, and Professor Jean-Noël Fabiani, chair of the history of medicine department in the same institution, for their generous assistance in the course of our research; also to Bernadette Molitor, librarian in the Faculté de Médecine de Paris, and Martine Bui and Sophie Richier at the Archives de l'Assistance Publique in Paris, for their competent and diligent work.

Special thanks, too, to Dr. Olivier Sarazin and Dr. Christian Reignier for all their help, and to Philippe Martinez, with whom we had productive conversations as we began the writing of the book.

Thanks, finally, to all our friends at the Institut Alfred Fournier in Paris. And to Malcolm DeBevoise for his care and thoroughness in translating the French edition.

—Bruno Halioua
—Bernard Ziskind

Index

Bronchopulmonary disease, 143–144
Brooklyn papyrus, 35, 38–39, 141, 143, 193; "Antivenomous Medications and Medicinal Treatments," 143
Brothwell, Don, 55, 110, 155
Brugsch, Heinrich, 118, 189, 226n11
Bubonic plague, 203
Bucaille, Maurice, 55
Bu-Hakah, Rayana, 203
Burial chambers, 10, 20
Burning bush, 198
Burns, 160
Byblos, 45

Cairo papyri, 24, 194
Calamine, 81
Cambyses, 23, 179
Canaanites, 183
Cannibalism, 125–126
Carbohydrates, 64
Carbon-14 dating, 62
Carbon monoxide poisoning, 158, 164
Carbuncles, 39
Cardiovascular disorders, 100–102, 162–165
Caria, 183
Carinate thorax, 104
Carlsberg papyri, 70, 193
Carob, 163
Cartilage, 38
Cataracts, 100
Cauterization, 35
Cedar of Lebanon, 38
Celery, 86, 163
Chameleons, 159–160
Champdor, Albert, 1
Champollion, Jean-François, 2, 189
Charcoal, 165
Charmers, 7, 140
Cheops. See Khufu
Chester Beatty papyri, 13, 29, 93, 170–171, 193
Chest of Bubastis, 24
Chickpeas, 163
Childbirth, 73–75, 186
Children, 32; circumcision, 35, 90–92, 186, 222n15; honor from, 69; gender determination, 71–72; infant mortality, 75, 96; neonatal care, 75–78; newborns, 75–81; breastfeeding, 78–

81; expense of, 82; *saa* and, 82; coughing, 82, 86–87; bedwetting, 84; teething, 84–85; otorhinological disorders, 85–86; bronchopulmonary ailments, 86–87; demons and, 88–89; spells and incantations for, 88–89; *baa* and, 89–90; adolescent, 90–94; youthful excess, 93–94; hunchbacks, 103–104
Cholesterol, 64
Christian era, 126–127, 167
Chrysanthemums, 174
Chryssipus, 100
Cilician fir, 38
C. I. Milne ostracon, 195
Cinnabar, 37
Cippus, 142
Circumcision, 35, 90–92, 186, 222n15
Civic administration, 16–17
Clement of Alexandria, 184
Cleopatra (VII Philopater), 189
Clepsydra, 25
Clinical examination, 24–29, 141; pulse taking, 25, 72–73, 101; worksite accidents and, 130–133; herniated disks and, 135, 137
Clysters, 13
Cnidus, 184
Coachytes (keepers of the mummies), 51
Cobras, 141
Cockburn, Aidan, 64
Coffins, 46
Colds, 82, 85–86
Computerized axial tomography (CAT) scanner, 56–57, 218n13, 221n6
Constipation, 170–171
Construction workers: foremen, 128–129; sick leave, 129; physicians for, 129–130; ophthalmological disorders, 129, 133–135; surgery, 130–131; worksite accidents, 131–133; herniated disks, 135–137; tetanus, 135; scorpions and, 137, 139
Contraception, 175–177
Copper, 19, 37, 39, 139
Coriander, 163
Cos, 184
Cosmetics, 134
Cotton, 35
Coughing, 26, 82, 86–87